Clinical Manual
for Swallowing Disorders

Thomas Murry, PhD

Professor
Department of Otolaryngology

University of Pittsburgh
Pittsburgh, Pennsylvania

Ricardo L. Carrau, MD, FACS

Associate Professor
Department of Otolaryngology

University of Pittsburgh, School of Medicine
Pittsburgh, Pennsylvania

SINGULAR

TM

THOMSON LEARNING

SINGULAR

✴ TM

THOMSON LEARNING

Health Care Publishing Director:
William Brottmiller

Acquisitions Editor:
Marie Linvill

Development Editor:
Kristin Banach

Executive Marketing Manager:
Dawn F. Gerrain

Marketing Manager:
Kathryn Bamberger

Project Editor:
Patricia Gillivan

Production Editor:
James Zayicek

Library of Congress Cataloging-in-Publication Data

ISBN 0–7693–0065–0

Notice to the Reader

Publisher does not warrant or guarantee any of the products described herein or perform any independent analysis in connection with any of the product information contained herein. Publisher does not assume, and expressly disclaims, any obligation to obtain and include information other than that provided to it by the manufacturer.

The reader is expressly warned to consider and adopt all safety precautions that might be indicated by the activities herein and to avoid all potential hazards. By following the instructions contained herein, the reader willingly assumes all risks in connection with such instructions.

The Publisher makes no representation or warranties of any kind, including but not limited to, the warranties of fitness for particular purpose or merchantability, nor are any such representations implied with respect to the material set forth herein, and the publisher takes no responsibility with respect to such material. The publisher shall not be liable for any special, consequential, or exemplary damages resulting, in whole or part, from the readers' use of, or reliance upon, this material.

Contents

Preface

Swallowing disorders have surged to the forefront of the speech-language pathologist's caseload in hospitals, nursing homes, and outpatient centers. The clinician is often required to make rapid decisions for which there is no scientific foundation. Training and clinical experience often guide decision-making. Although these decisions may have a sound clinical basis, the effectiveness of swallowing evaluation and therapy remain in the clinical purview of the practicing speech-language pathologist and await extensive clinical trials. This text was written for the practicing clinician who makes daily decisions about the swallowing needs and safety of patients. By merging ongoing research and existing data into clinically useful information that can be accessed quickly, it focuses on the needs of individuals in clinical practicums and those who treat swallowing disorders.

Our experience gained from working together in a team format as well as conducting research in dysphagia and related topics is the basis for this text. While the speech-language pathologist is the focal person for this text, all rehabilitation disciplines are considered in the diagnosis and treatment paradigms. Since the practicing clinician is expected to be well-versed in the anatomy and physiology of the swallowing mechanism, this topic is not covered fully in this text. Other texts review the anatomy and physiology of the head and neck in detail. We focus on issues relating to the daily clinical practice of swallowing.

Chapter 1 presents the clinical arena of dysphagia—who has dysphagia and the indications for intervention. Definitions of key terms used throughout the book are provided. The importance of early intervention is addressed despite the lack of basic clinical research supporting many of the therapies used to treat swallowing disorders. The financial and psychological impacts of dysphagia on patients and their families are reviewed. The most current epidemiological data available is also given in this chapter.

Chapter 2 presents an overview of the anatomy and function of the swallowing mechanism. The phases of the normal swallow are detailed. The importance of the sphincter and propulsive musculature is explained. A description of the cranial nerves used in swallowing as well as their functions is provided. A table provides a diagnostic guide to the swallowing disorder based on dysfunctions according to the phases of swallowing.

Chapter 3 describes the disorders of swallowing. This chapter includes an extensive array of tables outlining risks factors for dysphagia and aspiration pneumonia, drugs that affect the ability to swallow normally, and an extensive list of neurological disorders that should alert the clinician to swallowing problems. Aspiration pneumonia is described in detail and patient groups at risk to develop aspiration pneumonia are described. The swallowing disorders associated with autoimmune diseases, esophageal disorders, infectious diseases, neoplasms, and neurological and neuromuscular disorders are presented in a format that offers the clinician information useful in the diagnosis and treatment of the swallowing disorders associated with these conditions.

Chapter 4 identifies swallowing disorders resulting from surgical treatments. With the popularization of new surgical procedures such as anterior cervical spine surgery, oncologic skull base surgery, and oral surgeries for lip, tongue, and palate growths, swallowing is affected on a temporary basis and often on a permanent basis. Indications for aggressive and conservative treatments for these problems are presented in this chapter.

Chapter 5 presents the various methods to evaluate dysphagia. A significant portion of the chapter is devoted to the bedside swallow evaluation. We have found this to be a crucial aspect of the subsequent testing and treatment of swallowing disorders. Moreover, our experience with the bedside swallow evaluation has led us to identifying the appropriate testing to be done subsequently and to obtaining the proper consultants to participate in the management of patients with various swallowing disorders. Nonetheless, the bedside swallow evaluation is rarely the only evaluation done when a patient presents with a swallowing disorder; therefore, we have outlined the most important clinical tests for diagnosing the cause of the swallowing disorder and when these tests should be ordered.

Chapters 6 and 7 review the nonsurgical and surgical treatments of swallowing disorders. While the focus of this text is the clinical rehabilitation of swallowing, we felt it necessary to include surgical management of dysphagia as it complements the conservative nonsurgical treatments. Chapter 6, which describes the advantages of current nonsurgical treatments along with their caveats, includes treatments for those patients who present with swallowing disorders resulting from surgery as well as those with swallowing disorders resulting from neurological disorders and neuromuscular degenerative disorders. Major techniques and their rationales are outlined in tables for use in the test. Chapter 6 provides a comprehensive array of treatment techniques in an easy-to-understand format for all rehabilitation specialists. Chapter 7 describes surgical treatments for swallowing disorders ranging from conservative procedures to help close the glottis to extensive procedures requiring complex decisions by the entire swallowing team.

Chapter 8 presents the most current information on nutrition and diets. A unique aspect of this chapter is the extensive explanation of the properties of liquids and foods that affect the ease with which they can be swallowed. Terminology associated with the science of rheology, which is the study of fluid properties, is provided and the applications of rheology to swallowing disorders are outlined.

This text does not contain extensive references. This was done in order to improve the book's clinical usefulness. However, a list of current references related to the materials in the text is provided at the end of the book.

By structuring the book into eight chapters, we hope to offer the practicing clinician easily accessible information. The structure of this book was developed from our day-to-day involvements in diagnosing and treating swallowing disorders with a team of individuals from the medical, surgical, and rehabilitative services in a busy inpatient and outpatient academic practice. This book was developed with a commitment to practicality and treatment of patients with swallowing disorders. We hope it will be useful in that way.

Acknowledgments

The authors acknowledge the following individuals who, by their direct or indirect contribution to the study of swallowing disorders, have contributed to the *Clinical Manual for Swallowing Disorders*. Previous research and publications by these individuals and others have established a strong relationship between the identification and treatment of swallowing disorders and the improvement of the health and quality of life of those patients affected by these problems. The authors are grateful for their leadership in this discipline.

Joan Arvedson	John Kirchner	Adrienne Perlman
Jonathan Aviv	Susan Langmore	Joanne Robbins
Michael Crary	Rebecca Leonard	John Rosenbek
Karen Dikeman	Jeri Lynn Logemann	Clarence Sasaki
Michael Groher	Bonnie Martin-Harris	Reza Shaker
David Eibling	Fred McConnell	Kurt Shulze-Delrieu
Marta Kazandjian	I.R. Odderson	Barbara Sonies

Clinical Arena of Dysphagia

INTRODUCTION

Dysphagia

Definition. The global definition of **dysphagia** is simply "difficulty in swallowing" This encompasses a person's swallowing of his or her saliva, liquids, foods of all consistencies, and pills. The swallowing difficulty may arise from mechanical problems of the swallowing mechanism, neurologic disorders, gastrointestinal disorders, or loss of organs due to surgery or trauma.

Related Terms. Related terms include

▶ **Aphagia:** The inability to swallow anything
▶ **Odynophagia:** Pain upon swallowing
▶ **Phagia:** Eating or devouring

Impact on Quality of Life. Any swallowing disorder eventually takes a toll on normal life quality through a number of ways:

▶ **Aspiration:** A condition in which foods or liquids pass into the airway below the level of the true vocal folds. Everybody experiences aspiration occasionally, but the normal individual has the ability to cough out the aspirate. When aspiration is frequent and/or significant, quality of life is diminished.

▶ **Aspiration pneumonia:** Pulmonary infection that results as a consequence of acute or chronic aspiration of fluids, foods, oral secretions, or esophagogastric refluxate.

▶ **Dehydration:** The state in which there are not enough liquids in the body to maintain a healthy level of fluids in the body tissues (i.e., negative fluid balance). Many patients with neurologic impairments have difficulty swallowing liquids and therefore reduce their intake of liquids.

▶ **Malnutrition:** Once a person is not able to ingest food safely, it becomes difficult to maintain proper weight and nutrition. Malnutrition can occur either due to the inability to ingest food safely or due to the reluctance to eat or fear of eating/drinking due to past swallowing problems. Malnutrition is often a presenting sign of a reduced quality of life.

▶ **Weight loss:** Weight loss can lead to weakness that is severe enough to affect the daily activities of an individual. When weight loss is ongoing, a swallowing disorder should be suspected. Any weight loss should not extend to levels that affect the quality of life, nor should it continue beyond a standard deviation of the recommended weight ranges.

Impact on General Health. The inability to swallow correctly may lead to a general health decline. This may be insidious or rapid and is usually, but not always, associated with other diseases. For those individuals with diseases such as Parkinson's disease, diabetes mellitus, chronic obstructive pulmonary disease (COPD), gastroesophageal reflux disease (GERD), or Charcot-Marie-Tooth disease, the concomitant disorder of dysphagia heightens the severity of the primary problem. With the onset of dysphagia, the body is frequently not able to cope with the primary disease. Moreover, the primary disease may be exacerbated by the dysphagia. The true level of dysphagia may be masked or hidden by neurologic or neuromuscular diseases. Therefore, in these diseases and syndromes, it is important to know the signs and symptoms of dysphagia and determine their level of severity.

Psychological Impact. Eating is a social function as well as a nutritional necessity. When a systemic disease is compounded by dysphagia, the natural social functions for which food plays a role are severely restricted. The person with a swallowing disorder can no longer blend seamlessly into those social activities in which eating is involved.

Financial Impact. The financial impact of dysphagia can be significant if there is a need for special foods, nutritional supplements, enteral or parenteral feeding, dysphagia therapy, special gadgets and appliances to aid in the preparation of meals, and or the need for personal assistance with feeding. Some or all of the expenses associated with these needs may be covered by health insurance. Nonetheless, the overall costs of all factors related to the management of dysphagia are substantial and may continue for extended periods, straining the economics of both the affected individual and society. Limitations brought by insurance capitalization or personal financial abilities often compromise ideal rehabilitation strategies.

The true financial impact of dysphagia remains unknown as research has not yet determined the true cost of aspiration pneumonia readmissions and the effects of a dysphagia rehabilitation program on reducing aspiration pneumonia. While the true cost/benefit values are not yet known for the early identification and management of swallowing disorders, conventional wisdom suggests that early intervention may prevent extensive comorbidities that result from the interaction of swallowing disorders with other diseases or disorders.

NEED FOR EARLY INTERVENTION

> *Not everything that counts can be counted.*
> —Denis Burket, as quoted in
> *Kitchen Table Wisdom*, R.N. Remen

There is only limited evidence that the diagnosis and treatment of dysphagia is efficacious from the standpoint of significantly reducing aspiration pneumonia. Most of the evidence that exists is based on studies of stroke patients. This limited evidence suggests that in the acute care setting, dysphagia management is accompanied by reduced pneumonia rates. Furthermore, the use of a complete bedside swallow evaluation (BSE) appears to be cost-effective in relation to the prevention of pneumonia.[1] Others have found dysphagia management to be effective in the rehabilitation of swallowing disorders in other populations; however, the lack of control groups, the effects of disease, and inadequate reporting of long-term follow-up limit the statements that can be made on the true effects of early dysphagia intervention for most diseases/disorders. Clinical observation, however, suggests that early, aggressive intervention is linked to improved quality of life, reduced hospital stay, and decreased incidence of aspiration pneumonia.

The lack of clearly defined research should not suggest that swallowing programs using bedside swallow evaluation or other tools, such as the modified barium swallow or the flexible endoscopic evaluation of swallowing, should not be continued. On the contrary, studies such as that by Odderson et al[2] provide strong arguments for continued early intervention in dysphagia. These investigators looked at pneumonia rates before and after initiating a bedside swallow evaluation program in a hospital setting. Aspiration pneumonia rates in stroke patients were substantially reduced after the program was initiated compared to before the program. Additional research is needed to provide further evidence of the effectiveness of protocols using bedside swallow evaluation, as well as multidisciplinary protocols that rely on instrumental techniques for the evaluation and treatment of the swallowing problem. It is important that programs in dysphagia intervention include a data acquisition format that offers an opportunity to assess their contribution to the reduction of hospital readmissions due to swallowing related problems.

EPIDEMIOLOGY

Dysphagia is a condition that can be caused by natural aging and by multiple disorders such as stroke, neoplasms, trauma, neurologic degenerative diseases, autoimmune disorders, and infections. Treatment modalities such as surgery, radiation therapy, and medications can also lead to dysphagia. Because of these varied and, many times, compound etiologies, it may not be possible to arrive at a specific incidence within any one category of disorder. This is especially demonstrated in patients with head or neck cancer who have a variable presentation of swallowing disorders before and after treatment. These patients may suffer from significant dysphagia at any point in the diagnostic or treatment phase but often enjoy a complete resolution of their dysphagia some time following treatment. Conversely, the typical patient with Parkinson's disease generally shows the opposite pattern, with the dysphagia becoming more severe as the disease progresses.

Swallowing disorders may arise as comorbidities of other disorders or as precursors to more significant diseases and disorders. Moreover, the incidence of swallowing disorders may vary depending on the procedure for examination. Table 1–1 shows the incidence of oropharyngeal dysphagia in patients who exhibited aspiration during videofluoroscopic examination.[3] The true incidence of swallowing disorders may be considered substantially higher if all examination procedures of swallowing are considered. When the swallowing disorder

Table 1–1. Incidence of oropharyngeal dysphagia in patients who exhibited aspiration during videofluoroscopic examination.*

Cause of Dysphagia	Number (%) of Patients	
Head and neck oncologic surgery	59	(36)
Cerebrovascular accident	47	(29)
Closed head injury	12	(7)
Spinal cord injury	10	(6)
Degenerative neurologic disease[†]	9	(6)
Adductor vocal fold paralysis	7	(4)
Zenker's diverticulum	4	(2)
Generalized weakness	5	(3)
Cerebral palsy	3	(2)
CNS involvement from AIDS	3	(2)
Craniotomy (for aneurysm repair)	2	(1)
Undetermined	4	(2)
Total	165	

*Adapted from Rasley et al.[3]
†Includes Parkinson's disease, motor neuron disease, and multiple sclerosis.

accompanies other medical conditions, the primary condition may be affected by the swallowing disorder. Conversely, a swallowing disorder may be the symptom of other neurologic disease or condition requiring treatment. Thus, the exact incidence of swallowing disorders remains unknown. In addition to these variables, not one of the tests used to diagnose dysphagia is 100% accurate.

Cerebrovascular Accidents and Neurologic Diseases

Cerebrovascular accidents (strokes) are the third leading cause of death in the United States. Approximately 500,000 new cases are reported yearly, and 150,000 individuals die of cerebrovascular accidents (CVAs) every year. Prospective studies have demonstrated an incidence of dysphagia as high as 41.7% in the first month after a CVA. The overall rate of aspiration resulting from a CVA is approximately 33.3%. One half of

Table I–2. Epidemiological data from the published literature: Neurologic Diseases and the Associated Rate of Dysphagia (Ref I).

Disease	Prevalence (per 100,000)	Incidence (per 100,000)	Study
Stroke	NA*	145 289	Brown, Whisnant, Sicks et al, 1996: Modan and Wagener, 1992
Parkinson's Disease	106.9	13	Mayeux, Marder, Cote et al, 1995
Alzheimer's Disease	259.8	NR*	Beard, Kokmen, Offord et al, 1991
Multiple Sclerosis	170.8	NR	Wynn, Rodriquez, O=Fallon et al, 1990
Motor Neuron Disease	170.8	6.2	Lilienfeld, Sprafka, Pham et al, 1991
Amyotropic Lateral Sclerosis	NR	1.8	McGuire, Longstreth, Koepsell et al, 1996
Progressive Supranuclear Palsy	1.39	1.1	Golbe, Davis, Schoenberg et al, 1998; Bower, Maraganore, McDonnell et al, 1997
Huntington's Disease	1.9	0.2	Kokmen, Ozekmekci, Beard et al, 1994

*NA = not applicable; NR = not reported.

these patients aspirate silently (no obvious clinical symptoms or signs). As many as 20% die of aspiration pneumonia in the first year after a CVA, and 10% to 15% die of aspiration pneumonia after the first year following the stroke. In general, the larger the area of ischemia, the more significant the swallowing disorder. Although the site of lesion

Table I–2. *continued*

Reason	Diagnosed Structure of Dysphagia (%)	Study	Reason
Mayo Clinic Mayo Clinic seemed low: this provides an upper estimate	VFSS: 74.6 74.6 BSE: 41.7	Daniels, McAdam, Brailey et al, 1997; DePippo, Holas, and Reding, 1992	Median of VFSS studies Median of bedside swallow evaluation studies
Only number on general population that included elderly	VFSS: 69.1	Bushmann, Dobmeyer, Leeker et al, 1989; Fuh, Lee, Wang et al, 1997	Mean of 2 studies in which L-dopa was withheld
Only published number	VFSS: 84	Horner, Alberts, Dawson et al, 1994	Only published number
Only number; Mayo Clinic	NR	NA	NA
Only published number	51.2 (method not reported)	Leighton, Burton, Lund et al, 1994	Exam, not survey
Exam, not survey	29 (method not reported)	Litvan, Sastry, and Sonies, 1997	Only published number
Only published number	VFSS: 55.6	Kagel and Leopold, 1992	Only published number
Only published number	VFSS: 100		

does not always correlate with the type and severity of the swallowing disorder, brainstem strokes produce dysphagia more frequently than cortical strokes. Table 1–2 shows the epidemiological data recently obtained from the Agency for Health Care Policy and Research (AHCPR) for neurologic diseases including stroke.

Dementia

Dysphagia is prevalent in patients with dementia. Normal swallowing function is found in only 7% of these patients, according to videofluoroscopic reports. This group of patients is the most difficult to assess with any type of functional study due to their dementia. Similarly, the effectiveness of therapeutic maneuvers that require patient cooperation is also low. Non-oral nutrition alternatives must be considered early in the management of demented patients with dysphagia. Recurrence of aspiration pneumonia, continued weight loss, and/or refusal to eat are key indications for non-oral nutrition alternatives.

Elderly Population

Seventy to ninety percent of elderly patients, even those without known neurologic disease, have some degree of swallowing dysfunction, if not true dysphagia. Objective functional tests are necessary to rule out specific diseases and assess the risk of aspiration. As many as 50% of elderly patients have difficulty eating, leading to nutritional deficiencies with associated weight loss, increased risk of falling, poor healing, and increased susceptibility to other illnesses. Weight loss, increased length of meals, depression, and general complaints of fatigue are often observed in this group prior to the diagnosis of a swallowing disorder.

Head and Neck Oncology

The presence of a tumor in the upper aerodigestive tract may affect swallowing by

1. Mechanical obstruction due to bulk or extraluminal compression
2. Decreased pliability of the soft tissue due to neoplastic infiltration
3. Direct invasion of nerves leading to paralysis of pharyngeal or laryngeal muscles, important for normal swallowing
4. Pain

All accepted treatments for squamous cell carcinoma—namely, surgery, radiation and chemotherapy—produce disabilities that are usually proportional to the volume of the resection and/or the radiation field. Surgery produces division and fibrosis of muscles and anesthetic areas due to the transection or extirpation of afferent neural fibers and/or receptors. Radiation therapy leads to **xerostomia** (dryness of the mouth), which, in many cases, is permanent and a main source of swallowing complaints by patients. Irradiation also produces **fibrosis** of the oropharyngeal and laryngeal musculature. Chemotherapy may lead to weakness, nausea, or reduced sensory processes and may add to immediate radiation side effects such as **mucositis,** the thickening of saliva and mucous in the mouth, pharynx, and esophagus.

Swallowing function after treatment appears to be related to both site and stage of disease. In general, patients with so-called anterior tumors, such as floor of the mouth or anterior oral tongue, have better posttreatment outcomes regarding swallowing than patients with posterior tumors, such as those in the oropharynx or hypopharynx.

Reconstructive methods also influence the swallowing outcome. Patients who are reconstructed with primary closure have fewer problems swallowing than those patients reconstructed with bulky insensate flaps.

Hospitalized Patients

The incidence of swallowing disorders in patients admitted to critical care units is increased by the need for endotracheal, nasogastric intubation and tracheotomy; by the use of sedatives or other causes of impaired consciousness; and by the overall debilitation common to most patients requiring critical care. Thus, acute care patients should be assessed for swallowing disorders within the first 24 hours of hospitalization. Furthermore, patients requiring mechanical ventilation are at higher risk for aspiration pneumonia. The mortality of nosocomial pneumonia is estimated at between 20% to 50% for hospitalized patients. Hospital costs due to nosocomial infection generally exceed $10,000 per occurrence.

Nursing Home Residents

Studies carried out in nursing homes have demonstrated that 30% to 40% of the residents have clinical evidence of dysphagia. The prevalence of all types of pneumonia has been estimated to be 2%, although it is unknown how many of these patients developed pneumonia as a result of aspiration. The death rate for patients diagnosed with pneumonia in a nursing home and admitted to acute care centers may be as high as 40%.

Others

Patients may present to an outpatient facility with numerous problems that include difficulty or inability to swallow. Other swallowing disorders may also be identified when a patient is hospitalized for the care of other conditions. Table 1–3 outlines the most common conditions that may indicate that a swallowing disorder is also present. The true

Table I–3. Conditions that may lead to or be directly related
to swallowing disorders.

Condition	Type of Dysphagia or Disease
Congenital	Dysphagia lusoria Tracheoesophageal fistula Laryngeal clefts Other foregut abnormalities
Inflammatory	GERD
Infections	Lyme disease, neuropathies/encephalitis Chagas' disease
Trauma	Central nervous system Upper aerodigestive tract
Endocrine	Goiter Hypothyroid Diabetic neuropathy
Neoplasia	Upper aerodigestive tract Thyroid Central nervous system

Systemic	Autoimmune:
	    Dermatomyositis
	    Scleroderma
	    Sjögren's
	Amyloidosis
	Sarcoidosis

Iatrogenic	Surgery Chemotherapy Other medications Radiation

incidence of swallowing disorders in patients presenting with these
problems is unknown.

REFERENCES

1. *Evidence Report/Technology Assessment Number 8: Diagnosis and Treatment of Swallowing Disorders (Dysphagia) in Acute Care Stroke Patients.*
   Rockville, Md: US Dept of Health and Human Services, Agency for
   Health Care Policy and Research; July, 1999. AHCPR publication
   99-E024.

2. Odderson IR, Keaton JC, McKenna BS. Swallow management in patients on an acute stroke pathway: quality is cost effective. *Arch Phys Med Rehabil.* 1995;76:1130–1133.
3. Rasley A, Logemann JA, Kahrilas P, Rademaker AW, Pauloski B, Dodds WJ. Prevention of barium aspiration during videofluoroscopic swallowing studies: value of postural change. *Am J Roentgenol.* 1993;160:1005–1009.

2

Anatomy and Function of the Swallowing Mechanism

INTRODUCTION

Though a thorough discussion of the anatomic and functional aspects of swallowing is beyond the scope of this book, a brief discussion is provided to facilitate the understanding of the pathogenesis, evaluation, and treatment of swallowing disorders. The functional anatomy of the swallowing mechanism is outlined in Table 2–1. The central and peripheral key components of the swallowing mechanism are shown in Table 2–2.

NORMAL SWALLOW

Phases of Swallowing

A normal swallow consists of four distinct—although interrelated—phases associated with specific anatomic structures: **oral preparatory, oral, pharyngeal,** and **esophageal.** For the swallow to be normal, the anatomic structures must be intact and their functions must be appropriately timed in sequence with each other. This requires the integrity

Table 2–1. Functional components of the normal swallowing mechanism.*

Oral Cavity

1. Bolus preparation
   a. Teeth
   b. Tongue
   c. Gingivo buccal and gingivo lingual gutters
2. Tongue driving force
3. Closure of oral cavity
   a. Lips
4. Oral control
   a. Soft palate
   b. Tongue elevation

Oropharynx

1. Oropharyngeal propulsion pump
   a. Soft palate
   b. Lateral pharyngeal wall
   c. Base of tongue
2. Velopharyngeal competency
   a. Soft palate
   b. Lateral pharyngeal wall, posterior pharyngeal wall/Passavant's ridge

Hypopharynx

1. Muscular propulsion
   a. Pharyngeal constrictors
   b. Pyriform sinuses
   c. Cricopharyngeal function
2. Larynx
   a. Closure: glottis, ventricular folds, epiglottis
   b. Hyoid elevation

Esophagus

1. Primary peristaltic wave
2. Secondary peristaltic wave

*From Carrau and Murry.[1]

of both the motor and sensory nervous systems. Clinicians involved with diagnosing and treating swallowing disorders should be familiar with the basic anatomy of the upper aerodigestive system. The anatomy of the upper aerodigestive tract is shown in brief in Figure 2–1 and Figure 2–2. (For a full discussion of the anatomy of the head and neck, see Sasaki and Isaacson.[3])

Table 2–2. Oral and pharyngeal phases of deglutition, contributions of cranial nerves.*

Structure	Afferent	Efferent
Lips	V2 (maxillary) V3 (lingual)	VII
Tongue	V3 (lingual)	XII
Mandible	V3 (mandibular)	V (muscles of mastication), VII
Palate	V, IX, X	IX, X
Buccal region/cheeks		V (muscles of mastication), VII
Tongue base	IX	XII
Epiglottis (lingual surface)	IX	X
Epiglottis (laryngeal surface)	X (internal branch of superior laryngeal nerve)	X
Supraglottic and glottic larynx (to level of true vocal folds)	X (internal branch of superior laryngeal nerve)	X
Subglottic larynx (below true vocal folds)	X (recurrent laryngeal nerve)	X
Upper trachea	X (recurrent laryngeal nerve)	X
Pharynx (naso- and oro-)	IX	X (except for stylopharyngeus, which is enervated by IX)
Pharynx (hypopharynx)	X (internal branch of superior laryngeal nerve)	X

*From Aviv J.[2]

Oral Preparatory Phase. Lips, tongue, mandible, dentition, soft palate, and muscles of the buccal cavity are temporally integrated to grind and position the food. The oral preparatory phase includes a **transfer phase** during which the tongue arranges the bolus and moves it posteriorly to a position where it can be chewed. In the normal person, the transfer phase usually results in the food being placed in the region of the molar teeth. At this point, the **reduction phase** takes over and the food

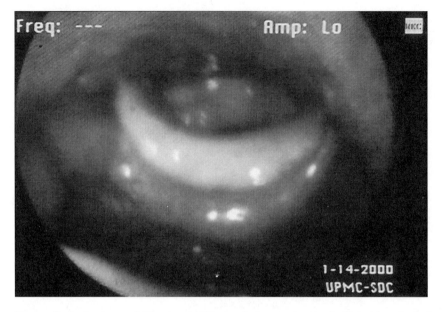

Figure 2–1. Anatomy of the pharynx. The oral pharynx is actually the midportion of the pharynx as the nasal pharynx is the superior extension and communicates with the nasal airway. The hypopharynx includes the base of the tongue, the pyriform sinuses, and the larynx and extends down to the level of the cricopharyngeal muscle. Reprinted with permission from Hollingshead. *Anatomy for Surgeons.* Philadelphia: Lippincott-Raven; 1982.

is chewed, ground, and mixed with saliva to form the bolus, which eventually is swallowed. During the oral preparatory phase, factors such as taste (via VII and IX), temperature, viscosity, and size of bolus (via V3) are sensed and appropriate lip, tongue, buccal, and dental manipulations are carried out to prepare the bolus for the next phase.

Oral Phase. The food bolus is transported via the action of the tongue and its interaction with the palate and teeth. The oral phase is primarily a delivery system. Contact of the back of the tongue with the soft palate retains the bolus within the oral cavity preventing early spillage into the pharynx. Once the bolus is prepared, it is positioned posteriorly on the tongue. The velum then elevates as the lips and buccal muscles contract to build pressure and reduce the volume of the oral cavity. The posterior tongue is depressed, and the anterior and middle portions of the tongue differentially elevate and begin the propulsion of the bolus to the oropharynx.

It should be emphasized that the tongue is the primary manipulator of food during the oral phase. Therefore, any injury or surgery of

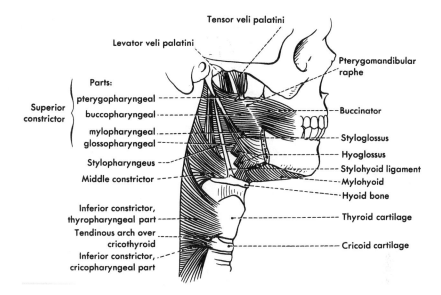

Figure 2–2. Lateral view of pharyngeal constrictor muscles and mandibular hyoid complex. Note that a portion of the superior constrictor muscle inserts on the pterygomandibular sphenomandibular raphe, which is continuous with the buccinator muscle anteriorly. The middle constrictor inserts onto the hyoid complex, whereas the inferior constrictor muscle inserts onto the thyroid cartilage. The cricopharyngeal muscle, the most inferior portion of the inferior constrictor, inserts on the cricoid cartilage and functions as the superior esophageal sphincter. Reprinted with permission from Hollingshead. *Anatomy for Surgeons.* Philadelphia: Lippincott-Raven; 1982.

the tongue affects the oral preparatory and oral phases of swallowing, either temporarily or permanently. Injury to the lips may complicate the problems in the oral phase. If lip closure and the maintenance of lip pressure is inadequate, the oral preparatory and oral phases of swallowing are affected.

Pharyngeal Phase. The pharyngeal phase begins when the bolus reaches the **anterior tonsillar pillars.** It involves the complex action of tongue elevation, velopharyngeal closure, elevation of larynx, and relaxation of cricopharyngeus musculature, all of which contribute to the movement of the bolus through the pharyngeal segment without penetration/aspiration into the airway. It is considered an involuntary phase.

Table 2–3 summarizes the signs and possible causes of dysphagia and its treatment according to the phases of swallowing. A detailed discussion of the treatment options is offered in Chapters 6 and 7.

Table 2–3. Diagnosis of dysphagia according to three phases of swallowing.

Type	Signs
Oral	Buccal pocketing, labial leakage
	Labored mastication
	Premature spill
Pharyngeal	Delayed swallow initiation
	Decreased laryngeal elevation
	Multiple swallow pattern
	Cough/throat clear immediately after the swallow
	Delayed cough, throat clear
	Change in vocal quality
Esophageal	Significantly delayed aspiration

Adapted from Simonian and Goldberg.[4]

Esophageal Phase. The **esophageal body** is a muscular tube extending 20 to 25 cm in length from its origin just caudal to the cricopharyngeus muscle to its termination at the gastric cardias. The esophagus shortens by 10% during swallowing through longitudinal muscle contraction. Although the primary function of the esophageal body is passage of injested material from the pharynx to the stomach, recent studies indicate that the esophagus is not merely a hollow passive conduit for food passage. Rather, it has several active functions for acid control and mucosal protection.

   Peristalsis or sequential contraction of the esophagus and relaxation of the lower esophageal sphincter characterize the esophageal phase of swallowing. The bolus is propelled through the esophagus by contraction above and relaxation below the bolus. This relaxation is referred to as **descending inhibition. Primary peristalsis** occurs when

Table 2–3. *continued*

Possible Causes	Treatment Options
Facial weakness	Oral motor exercises, surgical revision presents food to stronger side
Lack of dentition, poor cognition	Modify food texture
Lingual weakness	Chin tuck position, modify food texture
Poor oral phase, vagus nerve dysfunction, prolonged intubation	Thermal stimulation
Tracheotomy, discontinue Nasogastric, Tube suprahyoid muscle dysfunction, edema	Tracheotomy cuff deflation, d/c NGT
Decreased pharyngeal peristalsis/ contraction	Alternate liquid and solid swallows
Aspiration secondary to decreased epiglottic deflection, poor oral phase; tracheoesophageal fistula (rare)	Supraglottic swallow, modify food texture
Aspiration after the swallow secondary to pooling in the pharynx	Utilize dry swallow, alternating liquid and more solid swallows
Penetration to the level of the vocal cords, vocal cord weakness	NPO, modify food texture
Reflux, stricture	Medication, modify foods, GI referral

a swallow induces peristaltic activity, whereas **secondary peristalsis** refers to the initiation of a **propagated contraction wave** in the absence of a swallow. Initiation of secondary peristaltic contractions is involuntary and normally is not sensed.

Sphincters/Valves

Swallowing can be visualized as the passage of the bolus through a series of dynamic chambers. These chambers are separated by **sphincters** (gates) that help to prevent spillage of the material before the next chamber is ready to receive it. The sphincters also maintain a watertight closure that aids in building up the pressure in the paticular chamber to facilitate the propulsion of the bolus into the next chamber. The specific valving and sphincteric actions of the upper aerodigestive tract involved in swallowing are discussed below.

Linguopalatal Valve. Opening of the linguopalatal valve usually coincides with the onset of **pharyngeal transit** (bolus entry into the pharynx) and the initiation of swallow. During a swallow of more than 5 cc of fluid, failure to coordinate the onset of pharyngeal transit with the onset of swallow gestures can result in nasal reflux, aspiration, or regurgitation. In other swallows, however, particularly those associated with mastication, the linguopalatal valve may open repeatedly to allow small amounts of the bolus into the oropharynx and valleculae long before swallow sequence is initiated.

Velopharyngeal Valve. Failure to close the velopharyngeal valve results in leakage of the bolus or air into the nasopharynx and a diminished ability to generate appropriate oropharyngeal pressures to propel the bolus through the oropharynx.

Laryngeal Sphincter. Laryngeal closure occurs in a sequential fashion with approximation of the true vocal folds preceding false vocal fold approximation and, finally, approximation of the arytenoids to the petiole of the epiglottis. Failure to close the supraglottic and glottic sphincters during the swallow results in penetration or aspiration and in decreased ability to generate adequate hypopharyngeal pressures to propel the bolus through the pharyngoesophageal segment and into the esophagus.

Upper Esophageal Sphincter. The upper esophageal sphincter is a tonically contracted group of skeletal muscles separating the pharynx from the esophagus. The major component of the sphincter is the cricopharyngeus muscle. At rest, the sphincter is in a state of tonic contraction that minimizes the entrance of air into the gastrointestinal tract during respiration. Equally important is its function to prevent the entry of refluxed material from the esophagus into the pharynx.

The tonically contracted upper esophageal sphincter relaxes during the pharyngeal peristaltic sequence. The relaxation begins after the onset of swallowing and lasts 0.5 to 1.0 seconds. The onset of the **pharyngeal peristaltic wave** is marked by apposition of the soft palate to the pharyngeal wall, generating a contraction that lasts over 0.9 seconds and a pressure greater than 180 mm Hg. **Pharyngeal peristalsis** transverses the oropharynx and hypopharynx at about 15 cm/sec to reach the upper esophageal sphincter in about 0.7 seconds. After the relaxation phase, the sphincter contracts to generate a pressure that may exceed twice the pressure of the resting tone. This contraction lasts approximately a second prior to returning to baseline.

Discoordination of the pharyngoesophageal segment may occur due to neurologic deficits such as recurrent laryngeal nerve paralysis or brainstem stroke. Inadequate elevation of the hyoid-laryngeal complex and/or weakness of the pharyngeal constrictors also affect the function of the pharyngoesophageal segment as a sphincter.

Lower Esophageal Sphincter. The lower esophageal sphincter is a specialized segment of smooth muscle in the distal esophagus that relaxes with swallowing, permitting entrance of the bolus into the gastric cavity and preventing gastroesophageal reflux in its resting state. Gross and histological examinations of the lower esophageal sphincter have failed to identify a specific sphincteric structure. The lower esophageal sphincter muscle also possesses an increased sensitivity to many excitatory agents compared to that of the adjacent tissues, suggesting a greater influence on sphincter tone by nerves and hormones.

CENTRAL NEURAL CONTROL

Deglutition, the act of swallowing, may be initiated voluntarily or reflexively. Central neural control of swallowing can be divided in cortical and subcortical components. **Neural control** comprises a very complex interaction of afferent sensory neurons, motoneurons, and interneurons that control voluntary and involuntary/reflexive actions of swallowing.

Cortical regulation includes centers in both hemispheres of the brain with representation for the pharynx and the esophagus. These cortical areas have interhemispheric connections and projections to the motor nuclei of the brainstem. Bilateral hemispheric stimulation produces a greater response than unilateral impulses, and this response is intensity and frequency dependent. Both the motor and premotor cortical areas are involved with the initiation of swallowing or at least have the potential to modulate the contraction of the pharyngeal and esophageal musculature. Input from these cortical areas to the pharynx, however, seems larger than that to the esophagus. Similarly, afferent impulses from the pharynx, largely from the superior laryngeal nerve and glossopharyngeal nerve, have greater cortical area effects than those from the upper esophagus via the recurrent laryngeal nerve (e.g. swallowing reflex).

The *swallowing center,* identified as an area within the reticular system of the brainstem that comprises the ambiguous nucleus (cranial nerves IX, X, and XI), and the nucleus of the tractus solitarius (cranial nerves VII, IX, and X) interact with the nuclei of cranial nerves V, IX, X,

Table 2–4. Clinical results after cranial nerve injury.*

Cranial Nerve	Results After Injury
V. Trigeminal nerve (motor)	• Slight weakness in mastication
VII. Facial nerve	• Slight weakness in bolus control, weak lip closure
IX. Glossopharyngeal nerve (sensory)	• Failure to trigger the pharyngeal stage of the swallow, premature spill of material from the mouth into the airway
IX. Glossopharyngeal nerve (motor)	• Deficit from loss of function not great secondary to intact function of other elevators of the larynx
X. Superior laryngeal nerve (sensory)	• Loss of protective glottic closure and cough reflex protecting airway from material on the supraglottic larynx
X. Vagus nerve (motor)	• Inadequate velopharyngeal closure, nasal regurgitation • Incomplete clearing of residue in the hypopharynx, pooling of material above the level of the vocal folds, aspiration once the vocal folds open • Inadequate glottic closure during pharyngeal transit
XII. Hypoglossal nerve	• Bolus control problems • Crippled swallow if bilateral

*Adapted from Simonian and Goldberg.[5]

and XII. This collection of brainstem nuclei coordinates the **central pattern generator** (sequential or rhythmic activities that are initiated by neural elements without external feedback). Cranial nerve deficits cause changes in function that range from minor to life threatening. Table 2–4 lists the functional results after cranial nerve injury.

Impulses from afferent fibers arising from pharyngeal receptors that respond to touch, pressure, chemical stimuli, and water provide the means to elicit what A. J. Miller[6] has described as "the most complex all-or-none reflex in mammalian CNS, the pharyngeal swallow." Thus, sensory impulses from the pharynx serve to adjust the frequency and intensity of the contraction of the pharyngeal musculature and direct the protective reflexes of the laryngeal sphincter.

Similarly, at the cortical level, impulses from sensory receptors from the oral cavity provide the central nervous system (CNS) with information regarding touch, pressure, texture, shape, temperature, chemicals, and taste. Automatic adjustments and voluntary movements are combined to prepare the bolus before swallowing.

Both the cortical and subcortical pathways are important to the initiation of swallowing. Oral musculature is represented symmetrically between the two hemispheres, and laryngeal and esophageal muscles are asymmetrically represented. Most individuals, however, have a dominant swallow hemisphere.

Involuntary phases of swallowing are the responsibility of the brainstem. While these factors are somewhat understood, the interaction of functions between the voluntary and involuntary aspects of swallowing remains to be fully understood.

REFERENCES

1. Carrau RL, Murry T, eds. *Comprehensive Management of Swallowing Disorders.* San Diego, Calif: Singular Publishing Group; 1999:367.
2. Aviv J. The normal swallow. In: Carrau RL, Murry T, eds. *Comprehensive Management of Swallowing Disorders.* San Diego, Calif: Singular Publishing Group; 1999:24–25.
3. Sasaki CT, Isaacson G. Functional anatomy of the larynx. *Clin North Am.* 1988;21:595–612.
4. Simonian MA, Goldberg AN. Swallowing disorders in the critical care patient. In: Carrau RL, Murry T, eds. *Comprehensive Management of Swallowing Disorders.* San Diego, Calif: Singular Publishing Group; 1999 (Chapter 52).
5. Perlman A, Schulze-Delrieu K. *Deglutition and Its Disorders.* San Diego, Calif: Singular Publishing Group; 1997:354.

SUGGESTED READINGS

Miller AJ. *The Neuroscientific Principles of Swallowing and Dysphagia.* San Diego, Calif: Singular Publishing Group; 1998.

CHAPTER

3

Disorders of Swallowing

INTRODUCTION

Swallowing is a complex function requiring numerous muscle groups, six cranial nerves, and four cervical nerves. The nerves relay motor impulses and sensory data between the brainstem and the muscles of the oral cavity and pharynx structures. The muscles of the oral and pharyngeal region transfer data to the brainstem reticular formation, medulla, and frontal cortex via the facial, glossopharyngeal, and vagus nerves. A safe swallow entails the timely interaction of the latter nerves and muscles along with the muscles of mastication, which are innervated by the trigeminal nerve. Additional muscular innervation of the swallowing mechanism by the spinal accessory nerve aids in the complex motion of swallowing. Thus, swallowing requires an intact nervous system, and damage to any of these nerves or to the corresponding areas of the central nervous systems (brain, brainstem, medulla, cortex) has an effect on normal swallowing. This chapter reviews the disorders of swallowing found primarily in the adult population.

ASPIRATION

Aspiration is the entry of material into the airway below the true vocal cords. Aspiration can occur before, during, or after the swallow. **Prandial**

Table 3–1. Classification of prandial aspiration.

Aspiration Before the Pharyngeal Phase

- Most common type in central neurologic disease
- Due to loss of bolus control during oral phase or to delayed pharyngeal swallow
- Conservative management: thicken the diet, neck flexation during deglutition, supraglottic swallow, effortful swallow, thermal stimulation
- Surgical management: horizontal epiglottoplasty, tongue base flaps, laryngeal suspension

Aspiration During the Pharyngeal Phase

- Least common type of aspiration
- Due to vocal palsy, paresis, or incoordination
- Conservative management: vocal adduction exercises
- Surgical management: augment the paralyzed vocal cord

Aspiration After the Pharyngeal Phase

- Due to inhalation of uncleared residue at the laryngeal inlet
- Conservative management: thinning the diet, alternating liquids, Mendhelson maneuver, head rotation
- Surgical management: translaryngeal resection of the cricoid lamina, cricopharyngeal myotomy, laryngeal elevation

From Mendelsohn.[1]

aspiration is the result of food or liquid entering the airway. Table 3–1 summarizes the nature of prandial aspiration. While the neuromuscular pathogenesis is beyond the scope of this book, the most common conditions associated with swallowing disorders are outlined.

Factors that influence the tolerance to aspiration include the amount, frequency, and type of the aspirate and the oral hygiene, pulmonary conditions, and immune function of the host. These factors and their interaction with the neuromuscular system of the host are extremely variable. Thus, the definition of what constitutes "significant" aspiration must be individualized. Pulmonary syndromes that are related to aspiration are shown in Table 3–2. They include (1) chemical pneumonitis, (2) bacterial infection, and (3) acute airway obstruction. Table 3–3 describes the two types of bacterial infection associated with pneumonia. Patients may present with a wide spectrum of severity of aspiration syndromes. Multiple risk factors for aspiration are listed in Table 3–4.

Table 3–2. Pulmonary syndromes related to aspiration.*

Acute Respiratory Distress Syndrome (ARDS)

Interstitial and/or alveolar edema and hemorrhage, as well as perivascular lung edema. It may be caused by aspiration of acid refluxate.

Lipid (Lipoid) Pneumonia

Aspiration of oil-based liquid such as mineral oil given as a laxative, oil-based nasal spray or contrast material. In unconscious patients, especially those requiring mechanical ventilation, fever, hypoxia, and excessive tracheal secretions may suggest pneumonia. For patients requiring mechanical ventilation, placement in a semirecumbent position and active suction of the hypopharynx may reduce the risk of aspiration.

Aspiration Pneumonia

Aspiration pneumonia is usually polybacterial and is associated with a high morbidity and mortality. It is usually found in dependent pulmonary lobes.

Chronic Pneumonitis

Some patients do not develop a radiographic consolidate that could be diagnosed as a pneumonia but present with purulent, foul-smelling bronchorrhea, low-grade spiking fever, and varying degrees of respiratory compromise. A prominent bronchial pattern may be present in the chest radiogram.

*Adapted from Falestiny and Yu.[2]

ASPIRATION PNEUMONIA

Aspiration pneumonia is a bronchopneumonia resulting from the entry of foreign materials—usually foods, liquids, or vomit—into the bronchi of the lungs. There are typically three distinct pulmonary syndromes caused by types of aspiration.

Anaerobic pneumonitis in its early stages results in a low-grade fever. However, extended periods of aspiration lead to more severe symptoms such as fatigue, cough, and unconsciousness secondary to hypoxia. **Lung abscess** is an accumulation of pus that has been contained by a surrounding inflammatory process. Radiologically, it appears as a spherical-looking area with an air-fluid level often resembling a lung mass. **Empyema** is pus in the pleural space. If left untreated, empyemas produce destructive changes resulting in rupture of the pleural walls.

Table 3–3. Bacteriology of aspiration pneumonia.*

Community Acquired	Nosocomial Acquired
Anaerobes	**Anaerobes**
Fusobacterium nucleatum	Fusobacterium nucleatum
Peptostreptococus spp	Peptostreptococus spp
Bacteroides melaninogenicus	Bacteroides spp
Other Bacteroides spp	
Aerobes	**Aerobes**
Microaerophilic streptococci	Staphylococcus aureus
Streptococcus viridans	Enterobacteriaceae
Moraxella catarrhalis	Escherichia coli
Eikenella corrodens	Klebsiella spp
Streptococcus pneumoniae	Enterococcus spp
Haemophilus influenzae	Citrobacter freundii
	Acinetobacter lwoffi
	Pseudomonas aeruginosa

*Adapted from Falestiny and Yu.[2]

Table 3–4. Aspiration: Risk factors.*

Altered Level of Consciousness

Head trauma
Coma
Cerebrovascular accidents
Metabolic encephalopathy
Seizure disorders
General anesthesia
Drug/alcohol intoxication
Excessive sedation
Cardiopulmonary arrest

Gastrointestinal Dysfunction

Scleroderma
Esophageal stricture

Table 3–4. *continued*

Gastroesophageal reflux
Erosive esophagitis
Zenker's diverticulum
Tracheoesophageal fistula
Esophageal cancer
Hiatal hernia
Pyloric stenosis/gastric outlet obstruction
Enteral feeding
Pregnancy
Anorexia/bulimia

Iatrogenic

Prolonged mechanical ventilatory support
Tracheotomy
Anticholinergic drugs

Miscellaneous

Obesity
Neck malignancies

Postsurgical

Skull base
Head and neck
   Thyroid carcinoma
   Supraglottic laryngectomy
   Major oropharyngeal resection
Carotid endarterectomy
Anterior cervical spine fusion

Neurologic and Neuromuscular Disease

Cerebrovascular accident
Intracranial tumors
Amyotrophic lateral sclerosis
Parkinson's disease
Myasthenia gravis
Polymyositis/dermatomyositis
Guillain-Barré syndrome
Dystonia/tardive dyskinesia
Vocal fold paralysis
Progressive muscular dystrophy
Meningitis

*Adapted from Pou and Carrau.[3]

Aspiration pneumonia, like its etiology aspiration, may be difficult to diagnose even with invasive studies. In stroke patients, the overall debilitation, malnutrition, dehydration, and other systemic problems that accompany the stroke may precede the actual stroke, increasing the risk of aspiration pneumonia after the stroke. Other risk factors often present in patients with a stroke, as well as with head and neck cancer, such as poor oral hygiene with bacterial overgrowth or loss of sensory awareness that may occur after other prolonged illnesses.

The following include the most important groups of patients who are predisposed to aspiration pneumonia:

▶ **Altered mental status:** Nearly 70% of patients with altered mental status, regardless of the underlying disease, aspirate, possibly because of the inability to protect the airways and/or the discoordination between breathing and swallowing.
▶ **Prolonged mechanical ventilation:** Patients requiring prolonged mechanical ventilation and patients with a tracheostomy are especially at risk for aspiration. Aspiration pneumonia can occur after only two weeks on mechanical ventilation, and nearly 85% of these patients fail modified barium swallow testing with fluoroscopy for detection of aspiration.
▶ **Gastroesophageal reflux:** Acute findings in acid aspiration-induced lung injury include mucosal edema, hemorrhage, and focal ulceration followed by the development of focal necrosis and diffuse alveolar hyaline membrane formation.
▶ **Neuromuscular disorders:** These patients lose motor and sensory function of the upper aerodigestive tract, leading to a variety of disorders affecting cognition, coordination of reflexive actions, and loss of sphincteric and propulsive mechanisms.
▶ **Upper-aerodigestive-tract tumors:** Most of these patients experience some swallowing difficulty, either from the mechanical effects of the tumor, its interference with the sphincteric mechanism of the larynx, or due to the anatomic and functional changes produced by surgery, radiation therapy, and chemotherapy.

AUTOIMMUNE DISEASES

Autoimmune diseases are characterized by the production of antibodies that react with host tissue or immune effector T cells that react to self-peptides. Autoimmune diseases may affect swallowing by causing intrinsic obstruction, external compression, abnormal motility, or inadequate lubrication.

Crohn's Disease

Crohn's disease produces lesions throughout the digestive tract that vary in appearance, often resembling aphthous ulcers or cheilitis. Dysphagia is the most common presenting symptom of esophageal Crohn's disease.

Epidermolysis Bullosa

Epidermolysis bullosa is a rare disorder characterized by blistering of the mucosal lining, often elicited by minimal trauma, a variable onset. The oral cavity, pharynx, larynx, and esophagus may be severely affected, resulting in severe dysphagia. Pharyngeal and esophageal webs and/or scarring may be severe, mandating a gastrostomy or jejunostomy tube. Epidermolysis bullosa is often refractory to standard therapy using corticosteroids and dapsone.

Giant Cell Arteritis

Giant cell arteritis, also known as **temporal arteritis,** is an inflammatory disorder affecting large and medium size vessels. These arteries that originate from the arch of the aorta are the most affected. Pharyngeal, tongue, or jaw claudication may occur when the ascending pharyngeal, lingual, deep temporal, or masseteric arteries are affected. Systemic corticosteroids often resolve all symptoms within one to two weeks.

Mixed Connective Tissue Disease

Mixed connective tissue disease is characterized by clinical findings that may be found in a variety of autoimmune disorders, including progressive systemic sclerosis, systemic lupus erythematosus, and polymyositis/dermatomyositis. Similarly, the swallowing disorders described under each of these disorders can be a part of mixed connective tissue disease.

Esophageal motility is severely affected, and the majority of the patients have no peristalsis or low-amplitude peristalsis contributory to gastroesophageal reflux disease (GERD). Heartburn and dysphagia are present in up to 50% of the patients with mixed connective tissue disease. The treatment of the GERD may reduce the dysphagia.

Myositis

Polymyositis and **dermatomyositis** are characterized by inflammation of the skeletal muscle. Thus, muscles of the pharynx are often affected while esophageal smooth muscle is spared. A modified barium swallow frequently shows prominence of the cricopharyngeus muscle, decreased epiglottic tilt, and moderate to severe pharyngeal residue. Two thirds of patients with myositis have demonstrable delayed esophageal transit. Polymyositis and dermatomyositis are treated with corticosteroids.

Pemphigus Vulgaris

Pemphigus vulgaris is a rare, chronic intraepidermal bullous disease. Blisters most commonly develop on the soft palate but can occur anywhere on the oral cavity. Painful ulcerations, which often become superinfected, follow the rupturing of the blisters. Ulcerations heal by secondary intention, often leading to scarring. Distal involvement of the pharynx, larynx, and esophagus is possible and may account for the dysphagia in some patients.

Pemphigoid

Cicatricial pemphigoid is a chronic blistering disease that affects the oral mucosa in almost all cases. Typical lesions are characterized by erosion of the gingiva and buccal mucosa and usually are not as painful as those associated with pemphigus vulgaris. As the targeted proteins are found in the basement-membrane zone, the lesions heal with submucosal scarring. Treatment of pemphigoid is primarily with corticosteroids.

Rheumatoid Arthritis

Rheumatoid arthritis (RA) is a chronic relapsing inflammatory arthritis, usually affecting multiple diarthrodial joints and present with a variable degree of systemic involvement. Women are more commonly affected than men, with a ratio of 3:1.

Rheumatoid arthritis is associated with xerostomia, temporomandibular joint (TMJ) syndrome, a decrease in the amplitude of the peristaltic pressure complex in the striated part of the esophagus (proximal), and cervical spine arthritic disease, all of which cause or contribute to swallowing problems. Rheumatic laryngeal involvement can result in cricoarytenoid joint fixation. Objective functional testing is necessary to determine the contributions of the oral phase and the pharyngeal phase to the swallowing disorder. Treatment of the dysphagia is focused on hydration and artificial saliva and/or pilocarpine for the xerostomia. Dysfunction from TMJ syndrome (i.e., trismus, mastication problems) is treated with nonsteroidal anti-inflammatory agents and exercises with mechanical devices. Laryngeal closure exercises may also be useful.

Sarcoidosis

Sarcoidosis is a chronic systemic disorder presumed to have an autoimmune pathogenesis. Sarcoidosis may cause laryngeal lesions, extrinsic compression of the esophagus by mediastinal adenopathy, and esophageal dysmotility due to myopathy, infiltration of Auerbach's plexus, or granulomatous infiltration of the esophageal wall, which may produce long segments of esophageal stenosis.

Scleroderma

Scleroderma, or progressive systemic sclerosis, is a disorder characterized by progressive fibrosis and vascular changes. The most common and the earliest symptom in people with progressive systemic sclerosis is Raynaud's phenomenon, characterized by pallor and sweating of the fingers or hands that progress to cyanosis and pain. Dysphagia, which is the second most common symptom of this disorder, is usually first noticed while swallowing solids.

Dysphagia is most often due to poor motility through the inferior two thirds of the esophagus. The process starts affecting the Auerbach's plexus, which coordinates the esophageal smooth muscle. This is followed by a myopathy, which is then followed by fibrosis and strictures secondary to the noxious effects of gastroesophageal reflux.

The dysphagia can be minimized by adequate chewing and by reducing the bolus size. Esophageal motility can be improved by prokinetic agents such as metoclopramide or cisapride, the latter recently taken off the market.

Sjögren's Syndrome

Sjögren's syndrome (SS) includes dryness of the eyes, nose, and mouth. Xerostomia, oral pain, glossodynia, and dysgeusia are prominent features of Sjögren's syndrome. Xerostomia also increases the incidence of GERD, since it downgrades the ability of the esophagus to clear gastric refluxate and the bicarbonate antacid effect of saliva is diminished. Treatment is palliative and includes saliva preparations, pilocarpine, antacids, and H_2 blockers.

Systemic Lupus Erythematosus

Systemic lupus erythematosus (SLE) is an inflammatory disorder that is associated with a variety of autoantibodies against many different tissue components. However, the vast majority of SLE patients do not experience dysphagia and have normal esophageal transit studies. Dysphagia and/or chest pain is most often attributed to esophageal dysmotility associated with lower esophageal sphincter insufficiency and, thus, GERD.

Wegener's Granulomatosis

Wegener's granulomatosis is characterized by a granulomatous arteritis involving the upper and lower respiratory tracts, a progressive glomerulonephritis, and other extrarespiratory symptoms secondary to systemic small vessel arteritis. Wegener's often affects the hard and soft palate and may lead to extensive ulceration, an oronasal fistula, and velopharyngeal insufficiency.

Table 3–5. Possible causes of dysphagia in the critical care patient: Common signs and immediate trial treatments.*

Type	Signs
Oral	• Buccal pocketing, labial leakage
	• Labored mastication
	• Premature spill
Pharyngeal	• Delayed swallow initiation
	• Decreased laryngeal elevation
	• Multiple swallow pattern
	• Cough/throat clear immediately after the swallow
	• Delayed cough, throat clear
	• Change in vocal quality
Esophageal	• Significantly delayed aspiration

*Adapted from Simonian and Goldberg.[4]
†NGT indicates nasogastric tube.
‡NPL indicates nasopharyngeal laryngoscopy.

CRITICAL CARE PATIENTS

Patients admitted to critical care units often exhibit a variety of swallowing disorders. These patients, who are often elderly, are usually affected by multiple medical conditions and are frequently debilitated and deconditioned. They often need nasogastric or endotracheal intubation and/or mechanical ventilation, which contribute to the swallowing difficulty and to aspiration. Nasogastric tubes reduce pharyngeal sensitivity, predispose the patient to gastroesophageal reflux, and may produce inflammation and pain, which interfere with laryngeal elevation and increase the risk for swallowing difficulties. Signs of dysphagia, possible causes, and common treatments for the swallowing problems of this group are outlined in Table 3–5.

The diagnosis and treatment of swallowing disorders in these patients is complex and commonly limited by their primary condition or by the treatments that they are receiving. The minimum requirements for a patient to actively participate in the dysphagia evaluation

Table 3–5. *continued*

Possible Causes	Treatment Options
• Facial weakness • Surgical revision • Lack of dentition, poor cognition • Lingual weakness	• Oral motor exercises • Present food to stronger side • Modify food texture • Chin tuck position • Modify food texture
• Poor oral phase, vagus nerve dysfunction, prolonged intubation • Tracheotomy, discontinue NGT,[†] suprahyoid muscle dysfunction, edema • Decreased pharyngeal peristalsis/ contraction • Aspiration secondary to decreased epiglottic deflection, poor oral phase; tracheoesophageal fistula (rare) • Aspiration after the swallow secondary to pooling in the pharynx • Penetration to the level of the vocal cords	• Thermal stimulation • Tracheotomy cuff deflation, nasogastric tube • Alternate liquid and solid swallows • Supraglottic swallow • Modify food texture • Utilize dry swallow, alternating liquid and more solid swallows • Modify food texture • NPL[‡]
• Reflux, stricture	• Medication, modify foods, GI referral

process include the ability to maintain alertness, follow basic commands, and, ideally, to be 24 hours postextubation or 48 hours post-
tracheotomy. Swallowing evaluation in orally or nasally intubated
patients is usually deferred, although possible in selected cases (e.g.,
young patients with normal upper aerodigestive tract).

ESOPHAGEAL DISORDERS

Cancer

The most common manifestation of esophageal cancer is progressive
dysphagia. Other symptoms include odynophagia, regurgitation,
weight loss, and aspiration pneumonia.

The barium swallow esophagogram is the preferred diagnostic
tool and serves as a "road map" of the esophagus, providing information on the site of luminal narrowing, the degree and length of obstruction, and the presence of concomitant tracheoesophageal fistula.

The primary methods for palliating dysphagia involve endoscopic
techniques. Endoscopic modalities include the ablation of the tumor
using Nd:YAG laser or bipolar electrocautery, photodynamic therapy,
balloon dilatation, placement of expandable metal stents, and endo-
esophageal brachytherapy.

One of the simplest, but least effective, methods of endoscopic palliation is balloon dilatation. Dilatation is simple, relatively inexpensive,
and easy to perform. However, it involves the risk of perforation, and
the benefits are short-lived.

In one large series, Nd:YAG was used as a palliative treatment for
malignant dysphagia in 224 patients over a period of 8 years. The
esophageal lumen was successfully reopened in 98.2%, and 93.7% were
able to ingest at least semisolids following the therapy. **Photodynamic
therapy** is a relatively new modality approved by the Food and Drug
Administration for palliation of obstructive esophageal carcinoma.

External beam radiation therapy has been one of the most common approaches in the management of obstructing esophageal cancer.
Brachytherapy involves applying a radioactive source close to the
tumor to maximize the delivery of radiation while minimizing its side
effects.

Surgical bypass is an option for palliating dysphagia in a patient
with good performance status, for whom conventional palliative methods have been ineffective. Minimally invasive esophagectomy utilizes
laparoscopic and/or thoracoscopic techniques to perform the
esophagectomy. Alternatively, a gastrostomy or jejunostomy tube can
be surgically placed to provide enteral feedings.

Motility Disorders

Achalasia. **Achalasia** means "failure to relax." Achalasia is characterized by the degeneration of neural elements in the wall of the esophagus, particularly at the LES. The distal segment of the esophagus tapers, giving the appearance of a "bird's beak" (Figure 3–1). The diagnosis of achalasia, however, is confirmed manometrically with esophageal manometry studies, which are discussed in Chapter 5.

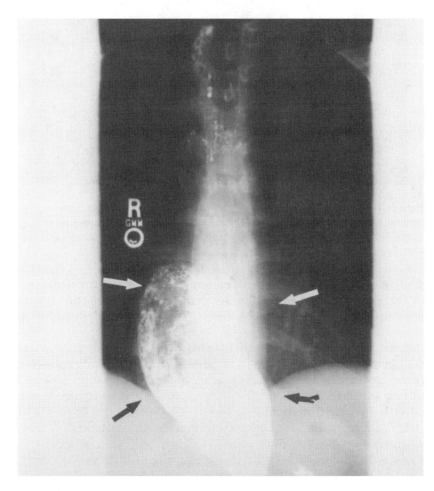

Figure 3–1. This barium esophagogram allows easy delineation of the dilated esophagus as marked by the arrows. (*continued*)

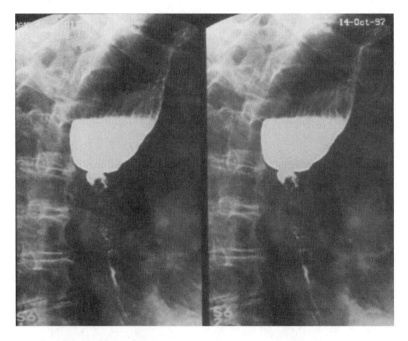

Figure 3–1. *continued.* The distal segment narrows at the lower esophageal sphincter with the appearance of a "bird's beak." Adapted from Padda S, Young MA. Chapter 27. In: Carrau RL, Murry T, eds. *Comprehensive Management of Swallowing Disorders.* San Diego, Calif: Singular Publishing Group; 1998:188.

Curling. **Curling** is an alteration in esophageal motility frequently seen in elderly individuals. Curling represents tertiary contractions, which are nonpropulsive.

Diffuse Esophageal Spasm. **Diffuse esophageal spasm** is characterized by intermittent dysphagia, chest pain, and repetitive contractions of the esophagus. Dysphagia is present in 30% to 60% of patients with diffuse esophageal spasm. Clinically, dysphagia is intermittent, with severity varying from mild to severe.

The distorted radiographic appearance of the esophagus is that of a "corkscrew" or of a "rosary bead" (Figure 3–2). Nonperistaltic or simultaneous contractions following a majority of the swallows are the most reliable criteria in the definition of diffuse esophageal spasm.

Nonspecific Esophageal Motility Disorders. **Nonspecific esophageal motility disorders** may be found during esophageal manometry in patients with dysphagia who have no evidence of other systemic diseases. Patients with nonspecific esophageal motility disorders constitute

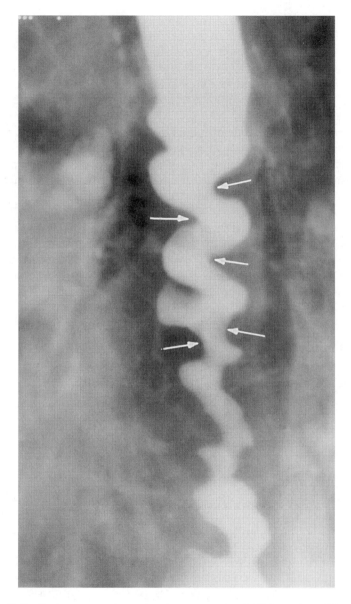

Figure 3–2. Corkscrew esophagus (tertiary contractions). Oblique view of the thoracic esophagus shows irregularly spaced contractions (*arrows*) causing indentations of the thoracic esophagus. At fluoroscopy, this was transient but recurred and the bolus was ineffectively propelled through the thoracic esophagus. This elderly woman complained of substernal dysphagia. Adapted from Weissman JL. Chapter 11. In: Carrau RL, Murry T, eds. *Comprehensive Management of Swallowing Disorders.* San Diego, Calif: Singular Publishing Group; 1998:73.

approximately 25% to 50% of the abnormal motility studies performed during the evaluation of chest pain.

Systemic diseases such as diabetes mellitus, amyloidosis, and, most notable, progressive systemic sclerosis (PSS) can produce esophageal dysmotility and dysphagia. An estimated 50% to 90% of patients with PSS have esophageal involvement.

Presbyesophagus. **Presbyesophagus** describes esophageal dysmotility associated with the normal aging process. This may include muscular weakness, muscular atrophy, or reduced speed of movement. This diagnosis is often specified in greater detail following appropriate assessment of neurologic instrumental testing.

Diverticula. Esophageal **diverticula** are outpouchings of one or more layers of the esophageal wall. These diverticula occur (1) immediately above the upper esophageal sphincter (Zenker's diverticulum); (2) near the mid point of the esophagus (traction diverticulum); or (3) immediately above the lower esophageal sphincter (epiphrenic diverticulum) or at the gastroesophageal junction (Figure 3–3).

Webs/Rings

Patients with intermittent dysphagia for solids may have esophageal **webs** or **rings.** Esophageal webs are reported in 7% of the patients presenting with dysphagia. A **Schatzki ring** is a lower esophageal mucosal ring, which is located at the level of the squamocolumnar junction (Figure 3–4).

Gastroesophageal Reflux Disease

Gastroesophageal reflux disease (GERD) is defined as the retrograde movement of gastric contents from the stomach through the lower esophageal sphincter and into the esophagus. A study that surveyed presumably normal hospital staff and employees found that 7% of the people interviewed experienced daily heartburn. The prevalence of monthly heartburn was estimated to be 36% to 44%. A randomized study of 2000 subjects demonstrated a prevalence of 58.1% of white patients with symptoms of heartburn and/or acid regurgitation. The prevalence of weekly or more frequent episodes of heartburn or acid regurgitation was 19.4%.

Persons with GERD frequently complain of noncardiac chest pain, regurgitation of gastric contents, waterbrash (stimulated salivary secretion by esophageal acid), dysphagia, and sometimes **odynophagia**

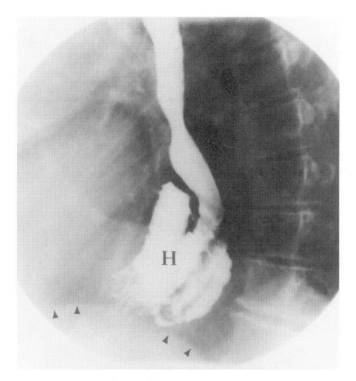

Figure 3–3. Hiatal hernia. Oblique view of the gastroesophageal junction shows a moderately large hiatal hernia (*H*) above the diaphragm (*arrowheads*). Adapted from Weissman JL. Chapter 11. In: Carrau RL, Murry T, eds. *Comprehensive Management of Swallowing Disorders.* San Diego, Calif: Singular Publishing Group; 1998:73.

(pain upon swallowing). Gastroesophageal reflux disease has also been associated with numerous extra-esophageal symptoms including pharyngitis, laryngitis, hoarseness, chronic cough, asthma, and pulmonary aspiration. Acid reflux induced symptoms referable to the oropharyngeal, laryngeal, and respiratory tracts are termed **atypical reflux** or **laryngopharyngeal reflux.** Table 3–6 describes the typical and atypical symptoms of the two types of reflux.

Some researchers feel that GERD may be the underlying etiology of **globus** (sensation of a lump in the throat). Gastroesophageal reflux disease was reported in 64% of patients reporting globus that were studied by ambulatory pH monitoring and has also been implicated in the etiology of oropharyngeal dysphagia, the difficulty in passing a food bolus from the oropharynx into the upper esophagus. It has been reported that 50% of patients with GERD experience cervical dysphagia at some time.

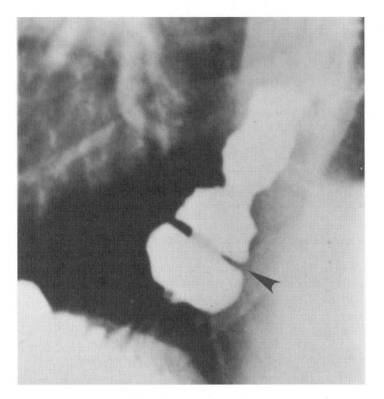

Figure 3–4. This barium esophagogram shows a typical Schatzki ring in the distal esophagus as indicated by the arrow. Adapted from Padda S, Young MA. Chapter 11. In: Carrau RL, Murray T, eds. *Comprehensive Management of Swallowing Disorders.* San Diego, Calif: Singular Publishing Group; 1998:192.

Table 3–6. Symptoms of gastroesophageal reflux.*

Esophageal	Extra-esophageal (Laryngopharyngeal)
Heartburn	Pharyngitis
Acid regurgitation	Laryngitis
Waterbrash	Hoarseness
Dysphagia	Globus
Odynophagia	Chronic cough
	Asthma
	Pulmonary aspiration

*Adapted from Levy and Young.[5]

Table 3–7. Substances influencing lower esophageal sphincter pressure.*

Increase Lower Esophageal Sphincter Pressure	Decrease Lower Esophageal Sphincter Pressure
Hormones	Secretin
Gastrin	Cholecystokinin
Norepinephrine	Glucagon
Acetylcholine	Nitric Oxide
Motilin	Pancreatic Polypeptide
	Intestinal Polypeptide
	Substance P
	Progesterone
	Cholinergic Agonists
	Cholinergic Antagonists
	Alpha Adrenergic Agonists
	Alpha Adrenergic Antagonists
	Beta Adrenergic Antagonists
	Beta Adrenergic Agonists
	Anatacids
	Barbiturates
Pharmacologic Agents	Diazepam
	Calcium Channel Blockers
Metoclopramide	Theophylline
Cisapride	Morphine
Domperidone	Dopamine
Prostaglandin F2	Prostaglandin E2 , I2
Diet	Fat
Protein	Chocolate
	Caffeine
	Peppermint
	Spearmint
	Ethanol

*Adapted from Levy and Young.[5]

Gastroesophageal reflux occurs through one of three mechanisms: (1) inappropriate or transient lower esophageal sphincter relaxation, (2) increased abdominal pressure or stress-induced reflux, or (3) incompetent or reduced lower esophageal sphincter pressures or spontaneous free reflux. Lower esophageal sphincter competence is the most important barrier to esophageal reflux. Transient lower esophageal sphincter relaxations are the most important cause of gastroesophageal reflux, both in healthy individuals and in patients with esophagitis. Table 3–7 summarizes the protective and injurious determinants of acid reflux.

Table 3–8. Determinants of reflux injury.*

Protective

Competency of anti reflux barrier
  Lower esophageal sphincter
  Upper esophageal sphincter
Esophageal acid clearance
  Esophageal motility
  Saliva
Epithelial tissue resistance

Injurious

Reflux constituents
  Acid
  Pepsin
  Bile

*Adapted from Levy and Young.[5]

Acid, pepsin, and bile acids are the active components of the refluxate contributing to GERD, as they are potentially damaging to the esophageal mucosa and submucosa (Table 3–8). The degree of mucosal damage by hydrogen seems to be potentiated by adding pepsin to the reflux material. The amount of time that the refluxed material is in contact with the esophageal mucosa might be a determining factor in the formation of esophagitis.

Upper esophageal sphincter dysfunction may contribute to the extra-esophageal disorders of GERD. Dysfunction of the cricopharyngeus muscle has been implicated in the development of Zenker's diverticula. **Zenker's diverticula** are formed by the herniation of the posterior hypopharyngeal mucosa between fibers of the inferior constrictor and cricopharyngeus muscles.

Barrett's Esophagus

Barrett's esophagus, a compensatory change in the esophageal mucosa from squamous to specialized intestinal epithelium, occurs in up to 10% to 15% of patients with atypical presentations of GERD.

INFECTIOUS DISEASES

Oral Cavity/Oropharynx

Bacterial infections of the oropharynx that result in dysphagia include tonsillitis, pharyngitis, and abscesses that may be associated with primary mucosal or lymphoid inflammation that causes pain and odynophagia. *Candida* infection may also involve the oral cavity and the oropharynx in both immunocompetent and immunocompromised individuals. It is more common, however, in the latter group of patients and in those who require prolonged treatment with broad spectrum antibiotics. The presence of oral cavity infectious diseases contribute to aspiration pneumonia and must be treated effectively.

Esophagus

Primary esophageal infections are unusual in the general population. When they arise, these are typically due to *Candida* or herpes simplex virus. Esophagitis, however, is a major cause of morbidity in individuals with impaired immunity caused by human immunodeficiency virus (HIV) infection, chemotherapy, and solid organ or bone marrow transplantation.

Chagas' Disease

Chagas' disease is a parasitic infectious disease that leads to achalasia. Chagas' disease, endemic in the Amazon basin, is caused by *Trypanosoma cruzi*, a parasite that destroys the parasympathetic innervation, leading to achalasia that, in severe cases, results in megaesophagus.

Deep Neck Infections

Deep neck infections are typically polymicrobial. In addition to symptoms of the primary infection site, patients may present with dysphagia, odynophagia, drooling, fever, chills, neck stiffness, and swelling. Treatment includes empiric therapy with broad spectrum agents, airway protection, and, often, surgical drainage.

Laryngeal Infections

Adult epiglottitis may cause life-threatening supraglottic edema that can progress to a delay in diagnosis and treatment. Common symptoms of supraglottic infection include a sore throat that is out of proportion to the findings of a pharyngeal examination, dysphagia, and odynophagia.

MEDICATIONS

The effects of medications are influenced by sex, age, body size, metabolic status, individual biological response, and concurrent use of other medications. A variety of medications, including those obtained over-the-counter and those medically prescribed, affect swallowing, impairing consciousness, coordination, motor and sensitivity functions, and the lubrication of the upper aerodigestive tract (see Table 3–9).

Analgesics

Salicylates (aspirin) and nonsteroidal anti-inflammatory agents cause ulceration of the mouth, throat burning, mucosal hemorrhage, glossitis, and dry mouth.

Antibiotics

Side effects such as **glossitis, stomatitis,** and **esophagitis** have been described for penicillin, erythromycin, chloramphenicol, and the tetracyclines. Sulfa can cause a Stevens-Johnson type reaction resulting in extensive mucosal ulceration and glossitis. Aminoglycosides can increase Parkinsonian symptoms of weakness.

Antituberculous medications such as isoniazid, rifampin, ethambutol, and cycloserine can cause confusion, disorientation, and dysarthria. Antiviral agents such as acyclovir, amantadine, gancyclovir, and vidarabine can indirectly cause dysphagia with confusion, asthenia, and lingual facial dyskinesia. Amantadine can cause severe xerostomia and xerophonia in some patients. Zidovudine (AZT®) causes dysphagia in approximately 5% to 10% of patients and tongue edema in 5% of patients. Chloroquine (Plaquenil®) can cause stomatitis.

Antihistamines

Antihistamines (H1-receptor antagonists) are commonly used to treat allergies. However, because of their anticholinergic side effects, this class of medications commonly exert a drying effect over the aerodigestive tract mucosa causing difficulty in gastrointestinal motility during the swallowing process.

Other common side effects include sedation, disturbed coordination, and gastric distress. Central nervous system effects include ataxia, convulsions, dystonia, and bruxism.

Table 3–9. Common medications affecting swallowing.*

Product Category	Examples	Common Indications	Possible Effects
Neuroleptics			
Antidepressants	Amitryptyle (tricyclic)	Relief of endogenous depression	Drying of mucosa, drowsiness
Antipsychotics	Haloperidol Thorazine	Management of patients with chronic psychosis	Tardive dyskinesia
Sedatives			
Barbiturates	Phenobarbital Nembutal	Treatment of insomnia	CNS depressant (drowsiness causing decompensation of patients with cognitive deficits)
Antihistamines	Cold and cough preparations	Relief of nasal congestion and cough	Drying mucosa, sedative effects
Diuretics	Furosenide	Treatment of edema (e.g., associated with congestive heart failure)	Signs of chronic dehydration (dryness of mouth, thirst, weakness, drowsiness)
Mucosal Anesthetics	Benzocaine Cetacaine Lidocaine	Topical anesthetics used to aid passage of fiberoptic nasopharyngoscopes, control of dental pain	Suppresses gag and cough reflex
Anticholinergics	Cogentin	Adjunct in Parkinsonism therapy	Dry mouth and reduced appetite

*Adapted from Perlman and Schulze-Delrieu.[6]

Antimuscarinics, Anticholinergics, and Antispasmodics

Antimuscarinics and **antispasmodics** are used for a variety of reasons such as bradycardia, excessive oral secretions, motion sickness, and diarrhea. They diminish the production of saliva and mucus. Salivary secretion is particularly sensitive to inhibition by antimuscarinic agents, which can completely abolish the copious, water secretions induced by the parasympathetic system. The mouth becomes dry, and swallowing and talking become difficult.

Prokinetic agents improve gut motility and speed gastric emptying. The two major drugs in this category are metoclopramide (Reglan®) and cisapride (Propulsid®) The former is associated with greater antihistamine-like side effects. The latter has since been removed from the market.

Mucolytics

Mucolytics can be used to counter the effects of drying agents such as antihistamines. However, no medications, including mucolytic agents, are a substitute for adequate hydration. Indeed, these medications are dependent on adequate water intake.

Antihypertensives

Almost all of the **antihypertensives** have some degree of parasympathomimetic effect and thus dry the mucous membranes. Hydration is the first step to improve swallowing when taking these medications.

Antineoplastics

Antineoplastics affect swallowing mainly through the mechanism of inflammation, sloughing, and occasionally causing superinfection of the aerodigestive tract mucosa. This effect results in mucositis, stomatitis, pharyngitis, esophagitis, and esophageal ulceration.

Vitamins

Overdosage of vitamin A causes hypervitaminosis A syndrome, which includes dermatologic, gastric, skeletal, and cerebral and optic nerve edema. Fissures of the lips, dry mouth, and abdominal discomfort can result. A similar stomatitis can result with vitamin E overdosage.

Neurologic Medications

Anticonvulsants. **Phenobarbital** is a sedative and anticonvulsant with side effects similar to the tricyclic antidepressants: dry mouth, sweating, hypotension, and tremor. **Phenytoin** (Dilantin®) adverse effects include central nervous system signs such as ataxia, slurred speech, incoordination, and dystonia.

Carbamazepine (Tegretol®) is an anticonvulsant used primarily for seizures. Digestive symptoms can also be serious such as glossitis, stomatitis, and dryness of the mouth.

Antiparkinsonians. **Levodopa** may improve all symptoms of Parkinson's disease including swallowing, but it can cause gastrointestinal discomfort, dyskinesia, and oral dryness.

Antipsychotics. **Antipsychotics** primarily work by dopamine antagonism. Commonly used drugs in this class include **haloperidol** (Haldol®), **chlorpromazine** (Thorazine®), **thioridazine** (Mellaril®), and **prochlorperazine** (Compazine®). These medications can have anticholinergic effects such as dry mouth, nasal congestion, and hypotension. Approximately 14% of patients receiving long-term antipsychotic medications will develop tardive dyskinesia ranging from tongue restlessness and disabling choreiform and/or athetoid movements that lead to significant swallowing and feeding problems.

Life-threatening dysphagia can occur after prolonged neuroleptic therapy. Neuroleptic drugs can induce extrapyramidal symptoms such as dystonia, akathisia, and tardive dyskinesia. Contrast radiography has revealed poor contractions in the upper esophagus, a hypertonic esophageal sphincter, and hypokinesia of the pharyngeal muscles.

Anxiolytics. Significant dysphagia can result from chronic use of **benzodiazepines.** Reported effects include hypopharyngeal retention, cricopharyngeal incoordination, aspiration, and drooling. Benzodiazepines can inhibit discharges from interneurons in the nucleus of the tractus solitarius or ambiguous nucleus, both of which are critical to the pharyngeal phase of swallowing.

NEOPLASMS

Neoplasia causes distortion, obstruction, reduced mobility, or neuromuscular and sensory dysfunction of the upper aerodigestive tract. **Exophytic tumors** interfere with swallowing principally by distorting or obstructing the aerodigestive tract. Tumors with an infiltrating growth pattern may cause reduced mobility or fixation of the tongue, soft palate, pharynx, or larynx (see Table 3–10). Tumors also affect swallowing by interfering with the afferent fibers (sensory input) from the mucosa of the upper aerodigestive tract by invasion and destruction of mucosal nerve endings or sensory nerves such as the trigeminal (V), glossopharyngeal (IX), and vagus (X) cranial nerves and their branches.

Table 3–10. Pathophysiology of swallowing in accordance with tumor origin and growth pattern.*

Tumor	Swallowing Pathophysiology
Intrinsic tumor	
Exophytic growth	Obstruction
	Distortion
	Anesthesia / hypesthesia
Infiltrating growth	Fixation
	Pain
	Trismus
	Cranial nerve deficits
Extrinsic tumor	
	Compression
	Obstruction
	Distortion
	Cranial nerve deficits
	Fixation

*Adapted from Falestiny and Yu.[2]

Neoplasms of the floor of the mouth, tongue, or buccal mucosa may by mass effect or by restricting mobility of the tongue and floor of the mouth impair a patient's ability to interpose food between the teeth. Tumor invasion of the dorsum of the tongue or involvement of the lingual nerve (V) may affect sensory input causing premature spillage of the bolus into the pharynx and, consequently, aspiration.

Tumors of the pharynx render an adynamic segment, thus interfering with peristalsis, or may interfere with the laryngeal elevation and cause mechanical obstruction. Tumors that invade or destroy the larynx may cause either an incompetent laryngeal sphincter or sensory denervation of the larynx, leading to aspiration.

NEUROLOGIC/NEUROMUSCULAR DISORDERS

Dysphagia caused by neuromuscular disorders is usually the end result of an impairment of the sensorimotor components of the oral and pharyngeal phases of swallowing. The onset, progression, and severity of the disease, as well as the symptoms, may vary. Table 3–11 summarizes the neurologic disorders causing dysphagia.

Table 3–11. Neurologic disorders causing dysphagia.*

Stroke
Head trauma
Cerebral palsy
Parkinson's disease and other movement and neurodegenerative disorders
Progressive supranuclear palsy
Olivopontocerebellar atrophy
Huntington's disease
Wilson's disease
Torticollis
Tardive dyskinesia
Alzheimer's disease and other dementias
Motor neuron disease /amyotrophic lateral sclerosis
Guillain-Barré syndrome and other polyneuropathies
Neoplasms and other structural disorders
    Primary brain tumors
    Intrinsic and extrinsic brainstem tumors
    Base of skull tumors
    Syringobulbia
    Arnold-Chiari malformation
    Neoplastic meningitis
Multiple sclerosis
Postpolio syndrome
Infectious disorders
    Chronic infectious meningitis
    Syphilis
    Lyme's disease
    Diphtheria
    Botulism
    Viral encephalitis, including rabies
Myasthenia gravis
Myopathy
    Polymyositis, dermatomyositis, including body myositis and sarcoidosis
    Myotonic and oculopharyngeal muscular dystrophy
    Hyper and hypothyroidism
    Cushing's syndrome

*Adapted from Perlman and Schulze-Delrieu.[6]

Evaluation of the cause of unexplained neurogenic dysphagia should include a careful history, neurologic examination, magnetic resonance imaging of the brain, blood tests (routine studies plus muscle enzymes, thyroid screening, vitamin B12 and anti-acetylcholine receptor antibodies), electromyography nerve conduction studies, and, in certain cases, muscle biopsy or cerebrospinal fluid examination.

Amyotrophic Lateral Sclerosis

Amyotropic lateral sclerosis (ALS) has an incidence around two per 100,000. Men are affected slightly more frequently than women, with onset around age sixty, although it may present earlier. Diagnosis of ALS requires the presence and progression of lower motor neuron and upper motor neuron deficiency. Upper limb muscles are affected more frequently than lower limb muscles, and bulbar muscles may be affected, leading to significant prominent dysarthria and dysphagia. Bulbar involvement in ALS is associated with a worse prognosis because of the higher risk of pulmonary aspiration and malnutrition. It is important to monitor the weight of the dysphagic patients and to begin discussions of percutaneous endoscopic gastrostomy (PEG) when the disease is diagnosed.

Lower motor neuron signs in ALS result from damage to the motor nuclei in the spinal cord (anterior horn cells) and brainstem motor nuclei. Upper motor neuron symptoms are due to damage to the corticospinal and corticobulbar tracts. Atrophy with or without fasciculations may be observed in the tongue and face. Spasticity or flaccidity may also be detected throughout affected regions. Patients with bulbar involvement are likely to show early lingual and labial weakness. The weakness progresses to the muscles of mastication and the intrinsic/extrinsic laryngeal muscle. The progressive loss of muscle function in patients with bulbar involvement produces difficulty controlling oral contents including secretions, food, and liquids, which may be observed as drooling early spillage of the bolus into the pharynx or pooling of residue in the gingivobuccal gutters. Patients are aware of these problems and respond to aspiration by clearing their throat or coughing when eating or drinking, suggesting a degree of preserved sensory functions. However, the effectiveness of the reflexive cough may be weak and eventually ineffective.

Dysphagia in the ALS patient leads to secondary complications, such as nutritional deficiencies and dehydration, which can compound the deteriorating effects of the disease, and therefore requires careful monitoring such as that proposed by Yorkston et al[7] (Table 3–12). At least 73% of ALS patients have dysphagia before they require ventilatory support, and an even higher percentage experience swallowing difficulty subsequently. Patients have more problems with liquids and large pieces of food. The ALS pureed or soft foods are much easier to swallow.

Drooling can be an early and disturbing symptom of bulbar ALS, often leading to social isolation. Many therapeutic approaches have been suggested over the years to reduce salivary production, including the tricyclic amitriptyline. Some ALS patients benefit from treatment with beta antagonists to help control thick secretions.

Table 3–12. Swallowing severity scale.*

Normal Eating Habits

10 *Normal Swallowing*
Patient denies any difficulty chewing or swallowing. Examination demonstrated no abnormality.

9 *Nominal Abnormality*
Only patient notices slight indicators such as food lodging in the recesses of the mouth or sticking in the throat.

Early Eating Problems

8 *Minor Swallowing Problems*
Complains of some swallowing difficulties. Maintains an essentially regular diet. Isolated choking episodes.

7 *Prolonged Time or Smaller Bite Size*
Mealtime has significantly lengthened and smaller bite sizes are necessary. Patient must concentrate on swallowing liquids.

Dietary Consistency Changes

6 *Soft Diet*
Diet is limited primarily to soft foods. Requires some special meal preparation.

5 *Liquified Diet*
Oral (PO) intake is adequate. Nutrition is limited primarily to a liquified diet. Adequate thin liquid intake usually a problem. Patient may force self to eat.

Needs Tube Feeding

4 *Supplemental Tube Feeding*
PO intake alone is no longer adequate. Patient uses or needs a tube to supplement intake. Patient continues to take significant (greater than 50%) of nutrition PO.

3 *Tube Feeding with Occasional PO Nutrition*
Primary nutrition and hydration are accomplished by tube. Patient receives less than 50% of nutrition PO.

NPO

2 *Secretions Managed With Aspirator/Medication*
Patient cannot safely manage any PO intake. Secretions are managed by an aspirator, medications, or both. Patient swallows reflexively.

1 *Aspiration of Secretions*
Secretions cannot be managed noninvasively. Patient rarely swallows.

*Adapted from Yorkston et al.[7]

In patients with prominent bulbar weakness, a palatal lift is sometimes useful to improve the velopharyngeal sphincter, as described in Chapter 6. Spasticity may complicate the bulbar contribution to dysarthria and dysphagia in the ALS patient. In occasional patients, baclofen can be effective in relieving some of the upper motor neuron impairment. Diazepam can occasionally be useful, but sedation and increased weakness limit its use.

Cerebrovascular Accident

Cerebrovascular accident (CVA) or **stroke** is the third most common cause of death in the United States each year. Between 30% to 40% of stroke victims demonstrate symptoms of significant dysphagia. Twenty percent of stroke victims die of aspiration pneumonia in the first year following a stroke. In addition, 10% to 15% of stroke victims who die in the years following the stroke die of aspiration pneumonia. **Cerebrovasclar disease** is the most common cause of neurogenic oral and pharyngeal dysphagia. Thus, dysphagia, aspiration, and aspiration pneumonia are devastating sequelae of stroke, accounting for nearly 40,000 deaths from aspiration pneumonia each year in the United States.

Although the correlation of site and size of the stroke with subsequent dysphagia is variable, the trend is that the larger the area of infarction, the greater the impairment of swallowing. In general, brainstem strokes produce dysphagia more frequently and more severely than cortical strokes. Robbins et al[8] suggest that the severity of dysphagia in patients with left hemisphere strokes seems to correlate with the presence of apraxia and the reported deficits are more significant during the oral stage of swallowing. Right hemisphere patients have more pharyngeal dysfunction, including aspiration and pharyngeal pooling.

Infarct size and distribution define the clinical presentation of the CVA and are dependent on the degree and site of interrupted arterial supply. In an MRI study of patients with acute stroke who underwent a swallowing evaluation, aspiration was present in over one half. Patients with only small vessel infarcts had a significantly lower occurrence of aspiration compared to those with both large and small vessel infarcts.

Dysphagia after unilateral hemispheric stroke is related to the magnitude of pharyngeal motor representation in the affected hemisphere. Patients with right hemisphere stroke show longer pharyngeal transit and higher incidences of laryngeal penetration and aspiration of liquid, as compared to patients with left-sided strokes. Lesions in the left middle cerebral artery territory are known to produce aphasia, motor and verbal apraxia, hemiparesis, and dysphagia. More than half of patients with bilateral strokes aspirate. However, dysphagia, with its attendant risk of aspiration, decreases over time in most patients.

Dysarthria and dysphagia, when associated with emotional lability, are suggestive of **pseudobulbar palsy,** a condition characterized by weakness of muscles innervated by the medulla (tongue, palate, pharynx, and larynx) because of interruption of corticobulbar fibers, as may be seen with multiple bilateral strokes.

Arterial supply to the brain stem is based in the **vertebrobasilar arterial complex.** The bilateral internal carotid arteries give rise to the majority of the anterior and middle cerebral blood supply. Each anterior and middle cerebral artery supplies the ipsilateral orbital and medial frontal lobe and the medial parietal lobe. Branches to the middle cerebral artery also penetrate the brain and supply the ipsilateral basal nuclei, internal capsule region, and most of the thalamus and adjacent structures. Each posterior cerebral artery supplies portions of the ipsilateral brainstem and cerebellum, inferior temporal lobes, and medial occipital lobes. Spinal arteries supply branches to the medulla.

Patients with posterior circulation strokes are more likely to aspirate and show an abnormal cough, abnormal gag, and dysphonia. Lateral medullary syndrome (Wallenberg's syndrome) is due to thrombosis of the posteroinferior cerebellar artery, which results in ischemia of the lateral medullary region of the brainstem. It differs from many other types of dysphagia in that the tongue driving force and oropharyngeal propulsion pump force are greatly increased, in part due to the failure of the pharyngoesophageal sphincter opening during swallowing.

Early screening and management of dysphagia in patients with acute stroke have been shown to reduce the risk of aspiration pneumonia, are cost-effective, and assure quality care with optimal outcome. The **Burke Dysphagia Screening Test** (BDST) is highly sensitive in identifying stroke patients at risk for developing pneumonia and recurrent upper airway obstruction (Table 3–13). Direct therapy programs for chronic neurogenic dysphagia resulting from brainstem stroke show that functional benefits are long-lasting without related health complications.

Myasthenia Gravis

Adult-onset **myasthenia gravis** is an acquired autoimmune disorder of neuromuscular transmission in which acetylcholine receptor antibodies attack the postsynaptic membrane of the neuromuscular junction. This reaction reduces the available muscle-activating neurotransmitter,

Table 3–13. The Burke dysphagia screening test.*

Patient Name: _____

ID Number: _____

Date of Evaluation: _____

1. Bilateral stroke   _____   _____

2. Brainstem stroke   _____   _____

3. History of pneumonia acute   _____   _____
   stroke phase

4. Coughing associated with feeding   _____   _____
   or during a 3 oz water swallow test

5. Failure to consume one half of meals   _____   _____

6. Prolonged time required for feeding   _____   _____

7. Nonoral feeding program in progress   _____   _____

Presence of one or more of these features is scored as failing the Burke Dysphagia
Screening Test.

Results: Pass   Fail

*Adapted from DePippo et al.[9]

Table 3–14. Diseases of neuromuscular junction.*

Myasthenia gravis

Eaton-Lambert syndrome (paraneoplastic impairment of acetylcholine release)

Botulism (food poisoning or intestinal colonization in infants)

Drugs (aminoglycosides, etc.)

*Adapted from Perlman and Schulze-Delrieu.[6]

producing rapid fatigability of all muscles. Myasthenia gravis is the most common of the diseases of the neuromuscular junction. Table 3–14 lists others.

Swallowing problems occur in approximately one third of patients with myasthenia gravis. Dysphagia is the usual presenting sign in neonates and in 6% to 15% of adult patients. Bulbar and facial muscles are frequently affected, causing dysphagia, dysarthria, nasal regurgitation, and weakness of mastication. Examination may show masseter weakness, bifacial weakness, poor gag reflex and palate elevation, dysarthria, or dysphonia. In addition, most patients have ptosis, diplopia, dysarthria, and dysphagia. Tongue weakness is very common when the bulbar musculature is involved, and the oropharyngeal transit time (posterior tongue) is especially affected.

Liquids may be swallowed easier than solids, and patients may fatigue with chewing because of masseter weakness. Patients typically do well at the beginning of a meal but tire at the end. Some patients deteriorate to a point where there is total loss of the ability to chew and swallow, causing aspiration. Patients should take meals when muscle strength is best, possibly one hour after medication such as Mestinon.® Compensatory training involves posture modification, alteration of food consistencies, frequent smaller meals, and other voluntary maneuvers designed to circumvent the health consequences of the oropharyngeal deficit.

Myopathies

Duchenne's Muscular Dystrophy. **Duchenne's muscular dystrophy** is the most common childhood form of muscular dystrophy, with an usual age of onset at 2 to 6 years. The inheritance is X-linked; thus, only males are affected.

Virtually all Duchenne's patients have severe dysphagia by 12 years of age. Episodes of aspiration pneumonia are common by age 18. For individuals with Duchenne's MD, deficits of oral preparatory and oral phases of swallowing, including increased mandibular angle and weakness of masticatory muscles, contribute to dysphagia.

Pharyngeal impairment in Duchenne's MD is associated with the appearance of macroglossia and weakness of the pterygoid and superior constrictor muscles. Weakness of lip and cheek muscles and tongue elevators may become more pronounced as the disease progresses. Pharyngeal swallowing reflexes are eventually delayed because of impaired elevation and retraction of the tongue. Aspiration of food and saliva, weight loss, and pulmonary complications ultimately occur as dysphagia progresses.

Facioscapulohumeral Muscular Dystrophy. **Facioscapulohumeral muscular dystrophy** is a slowly progressive, autosomal dominant neuromuscular disorder with onset in adolescence or early adulthood. Less than 10% of individuals with facioscapulohumeral MD have dysphagia.

Inflammatory Myopathies. **Inflammatory myopathies** involve the inflammation and degeneration of skeletal muscle tissues. Inflammatory cells surround, invade, and destroy normal muscle fibers, eventually resulting in muscle weakness.

▶ **Dermatomyositis:** Dermatomyositis usually presents with a rash characterized by patchy, bluish-purple discolorations on the face, neck, shoulders, upper chest, elbows, knees, knuckles, and back, accompanying or, more often, preceding muscle weakness. Dysphagia occurs in at least one third of dermatomyositis patients who typically present with oral dryness, delayed pharyngeal transit, and even aspiration.

High dose prednisone is an effective treatment for many patients. In addition, other nonsteroidal immunosuppressants such as azathioprine and methotrexate are often used, and even intravenous administration of immunoglobulins has also proven effective.

▶ **Inclusion body myositis:** Inclusion body myositis is an inflammatory muscle disease characterized by slow and relentlessly progressive muscle weakness and atrophy, similar to polymyositis, which follows. Indeed, inclusion body myositis is often the correct diagnosis in cases of polymyositis that are unresponsive to therapy.

Unfortunately, there is as yet no known treatment for inclusion body myositis. The disease is unresponsive to corticosteroids and other immunosuppressive drugs. Intravenous immunoglobulin has shown some preliminary evidence for a slight beneficial effect in a small number of cases.

▶ **Polymyositis:** Polymyositis does not have the characteristic rash of dermatomyositis. As with dermatomyositis, dysphagia is common in polymyositis and its symptoms also include dryness of the mouth and prolonged pharyngeal transit. Treatment is also similar to that of dermatomyositis and includes prednisone, azathioprine, methotrexate, and intravenous immunoglobulin.

Limb-Girdle Muscular Dystrophy. **Limb-girdle muscular dystrophy** is a slowly progressive form of muscular dystrophy with both autosomal recessive and dominant forms. Males and females are equally affected, with the usual onset in adolescence or early adulthood. Swallowing abnormalities are demonstrated in up to a third of patients, who show dysfunction of the pharyngeal muscles.

Myotonic Dystrophy. **Myotonic dystrophy** is an autosomal dominant disorder that results in skeletal muscle weakness and wasting, myotonia, and numerous nonmuscular manifestations including frontal balding, cataracts, gonadal dysfunction, cardiac conduction abnormalities, respiratory insufficiency, and hypersomnolence.

Radiological features of dysphagia in myotonic dystrophy include a marked reduction in resting tone of both the upper and lower esophageal sphincters and a reduction in contraction pressure in the pharynx and throughout the esophagus. Contrast radiography shows hypotonic pharynx with stasis and a hypomotility, often esophageal dilation, and gastroesophageal reflux disease.

Oculopharyngeal Muscular Dystrophy. **Oculopharyngeal muscular dystrophy** is a progressive neurologic disorder characterized by gradual onset of dysphagia, ptosis, and facial weakness. Oculopharyngeal MD is an autosomal dominant disorder that affects both males and females, with onset of symptoms in the fourth or fifth decade. Dysphagia is slowly progressive and may be a presenting symptom before a diagnosis is made.

Both striated skeletal and smooth muscle are affected, leading to very low pharyngeal manometric pressures, cricopharyngeal bar, and low lower esophageal sphincter pressure. Cricopharyngeal myotomy is an effective treatment of dysphagia secondary to cricopharyngeal achalasia. However, a cricopharyngeal myotomy does not modify the final prognosis and is contraindicated in cases with weak pharyngeal propulsion.

Spinal Muscular Atrophies. **Spinal muscular atrophies** constitute a group of neuromuscular disorders defined pathologically by degeneration of the anterior horn cells in the spinal cord.

Swallowing difficulties occur in over one third of patients with spinal muscular atrophy. Bulbar and respiratory involvement is a prominent feature only in early-onset, more severely affected patients, with respiratory insufficiency, difficulty sucking and swallowing, accumulation of secretions, and a weak cry.

Parkinson's Disease

Parkinson's disease is a progressive degenerative disorder characterized by loss of striatal dopamine. Oral and pharyngeal dysphagia in Parkinson's disease is multifactorial. Prepharyngeal abnormalities, including cognitive abnormalities, drooling, jaw rigidity, head and neck posture during meals, upper extremity dysmotility, impulsive feeding behavior, and lingual transfer are common in patients with advanced disease.

Pharyngeoesophageal motor abnormalities also play a role in the dysphagia of Parkinson's patients. Abnormalities include limited pharyngeal contraction, abnormal pharyngeal wall motion, impaired pharyngeal bolus transport, and manometric abnormalities with incomplete upper esophageal sphincter relaxation. Dysfunction of the lower esophageal sphincter includes an open or delayed opening of the lower esophageal sphincter and gastroesophageal reflux. Other esophageal abnormalities include delayed transport, stasis, bolus redirection, and tertiary contractions.

Pneumonia is one of the most prevalent primary causes of death in patients with Parkinson's disease. The disease is characterized by a release of subcortical inhibitory centers within the indirect (extrapyramidal) motor system, which modulates motor function. This is thought to occur due to the degeneration and depigmentation of dopamine-containing neurons found in the substantia nigra and its connections to the basal nuclei. The result is depletion of dopamine in the caudate nucleus and putamen, causing a motor disturbance that includes, among other signs, rigidity and resting tremor.

Disorders of the oral phase of swallowing are common in Parkinson's disease. Excessive lingual rocking or pumping, incomplete transfer of a bolus from oral to pharyngeal cavity, preswallow loss of bolus containment with spillage into the pharynx and/or larynx, and swallow hesitation are seen. Deficits during the pharyngeal phase include pooling of residue within the pharyngeal recesses and delayed onset of the pharyngeal response, predisposing the patient to aspiration before the swallow. Reduced lingual range of motion and rigidity result in diminished hyolaryngeal excursion, producing inadequate or incomplete distension of the upper esophageal segment, and incomplete airway closure with aspiration. Esophageal motor abnormalities are also commonly detected in Parkinson's patients.

Cricopharyngeal myotomy improves swallowing in Parkinson's patients with coexisting Zenker's diverticula but is not recommended to treat other causes of dysphagia.

Progressive Supranuclear Palsy

Progressive supranuclear palsy is a progressive degenerative extrapyramidal disease that often masquerades as Parkinson's disease. Almost all progressive supranuclear palsy patients show multiple abnormalities in swallowing, including uncoordinated lingual movements, absent velar retraction or elevation, impaired posterior lingual displacement, and copious pharyngeal secretions. Tongue-assisted mastication, noncohesive lingual transfer, excessive spillage of the oral bolus into the pharynx prior to active transfer, vallecular bolus retention, abnormal epiglottic positioning, and hiatal hernias are also noted in about one half of these patients. Unfortunately, progressive supranuclear palsy patients do not respond to dopaminergic pharmacologic treatment as well as Parkinson's patients. Likewise, their dysphagia is more life-threatening and resistant to treatment. Early and aggressive swallowing evaluation and treatment is mandatory in these patients.

Traumatic Brain Injury

Swallowing disorders in patients with **traumatic brain injury** consist of delayed or absent pharyngeal response, reduced lingual control, reduced pharyngeal clearance, and aspiration during and after the swallow. Cranial nerves can be affected due to skull base fractures and/or acceleration-deceleration injuries. Cognitive deficits in this population that may impact upon safe oral intake are disorders of attention, impulsivity, agitation, memory deficits, and reduced higher level reasoning skills.

RADIATION THERAPY

Dysphagia is a common side effect of radiation therapy for cancers of the upper aerodigestive tract and the head and neck regions. It is further complicated by the effect of surgical procedures that may be done prior to radiation. The etiology of dysphagia following radiation therapy is multifactorial and can be divided into acute and late effects. Acute effects present during and immediately following a course of irradiation, and late effects manifest themselves from several months to years after completion of radiation therapy. The acute phase of dysphagia is primarily due to radiation effects on mucosa (erythema, pseudomembranous mucositis, ulceration), taste buds (decreased, altered, or loss of taste acuity), and salivary glands (thickened saliva secondary to decreased serous secretions). Late effects include injury to salivary glands resulting in xerostomia and damage to connective tissue (fibrosis) resulting in trismus and poor pharyngeal motility.

Irradiation produces mitotic death of the basal cells of the mucosa as this is a rapidly renewing system (high cell turnover). During a standard course of radiation therapy (180–200 cGy/fraction; five daily fractions per week), there is a two-week delay from the start of therapy before the onset of mucositis.

Late complications involving the mucosa of the upper aerodigestive tract are primarily related to atrophy, manifested by pallor and thinning; submucosal fibrosis, manifested as induration and diminished pliability; and, occasionally, chronic ulceration and necrosis with resultant exposure of the underlying bone/soft tissue.

In humans, the parotid glands are purely serous, the submandibular glands are made of serous and mucous acini, and the minor salivary glands are predominantly mucous secreting. The normal human salivary glands produce approximately 1000–1500 cc of saliva per day. The parotid accounts for about 60% to 65% of the salivary flow, submandibular contributes 20% to 30%, and sublingual glands 2% to 5%. Irradiation of the normal salivary glands results primarily in injury to the serous acini with no significant effect on the mucous acini.

A decrease in the salivary flow can be detected 24 to 48 hours after initiation of standard fractionated irradiation, and it continues to decline through the course of therapy. In addition to the decrease in flow there is increase in viscosity, and decreased pH and IgA in saliva. Since the serous acini are primarily affected, the saliva becomes thick, sticky, and ropy, resulting in dry mouth and difficulty with mastication and swallowing. Most patients are unable to clear these thick secretions. These changes allow for an increased yeast flora of the oral cavity. The dose at which 50% of patients develop xerostomia at 5 years follow-up after irradiation was 7000 cGy.

Xerostomia results from permanent injury to the salivary glands. The most effective treatment for xerostomia is prevention. Once xerostomia develops, its treatment primarily consists of saliva substitute (water and glycerin mixture) and salivary gland stimulants such as pilocarpine hydrochloride, bromohexine, and anethole-trithione.

Pilocarpine is a cholinergic agonist that stimulates the smooth muscle and exocrine glands by its action on the postganglionic cells. This results in increased excretion of saliva and sweat.

REFERENCES

1. Mendelsohn M. New concepts in dysphagia management. *J Otolaryngol.* 1993; 22 (Suppl 1):9.
2. Falestiny MN, Yu VL. In: Carrau RL, Murry T, eds. *Comprehensive Management of Swallowing Disorders.* San Diego, Calif: Singular Publishing Group; 1999:385.
3. Pou AM, Carrau RL. In: Carrau RL, Murry T, eds. *Comprehensive Management of Swallowing Disorders.* San Diego, Calif: Singular Publishing Group; 1999:157.
4. Simonian MA, Goldberg AN. Swallowing disorders in the critical care patient. In: Carrau RL, Murry T, eds. *Comprehensive Management of Swallowing Disorders.* San Diego, Calif: Singular Publishing Group; 1999:367.

5. Levy N, Young MA. In: Carrau RL, Murry T, eds. *Comprehensive Management of Swallowing Disorders.* San Diego, Calif: Singular Publishing Group; 1999:179–180.
6. Perlman AL, Schulze-Delrieu K. *Deglutition and its Disorders.* San Diego, Calif: Singular Publishing Group; 1997:139, 322, 351.
7. Yorkston KM, Strand E, Miller R, Hillel A, Smith K, Speech deterioration in amyotrophic lateral sclerosis: implications for the timing of intervention. *J Med Speech Lang Pathol.* 1993; 1:35–46.
8. Robbins J, Levine RL, Maser A, Rosenbek JC, Kempster JB. Swallowing after unilateral stroke of the cerebral cortex. *Arch Phys Med Rehabil.* 1993; 74:1295–1300.
9. DePippo KL, Holas MA, Reding MJ. The Burke Dysphagia Screening Test: validation of its use in patients with stroke. *Arch Phys Med Rehabil.* 1994; 75:1284–1286.

CHAPTER

Swallowing Disorders Arising from Surgical Treatments

INTRODUCTION

Virtually all patients who are treated surgically for head, neck, or other disorders of the upper respiratory tract experience some difficulty in swallowing postoperatively. Dysphagia may be short-term requiring no special tests, diet modifications, or dysphagic treatment or may be long-term requiring the involvement of the entire dysphagia rehabilitation team.

ANTERIOR CERVICAL SPINAL SURGERY

Anterior cervical spinal surgery is a common surgical approach. Surgeons approach the spinal cord anteriorly with a cervical incision, mobilizing the laryngotracheal complex away from the great vessels of the neck and prevertebral space to visualize and repair the cervical spine.

Table 4–1. Complications of anterior cervical approach.*

Early dysphagia	100%
Prolonged dysphagia	5% to 11%
Hematoma	1% to 3%
RLN† injury	1% to 16%
SLN‡ injury	1%
Esophageal perforation	0.2% to 0.9%

*Adapted from Drennen et al.[1]
†RLN = recurrent laryngeal nerve
‡SLN = superior laryngeal nerve

Postoperative dysphagia is found in all patients who undergo anterior cervical spinal surgery. Although in most patients the dysphagia is of short duration, in 10% of patients it can persist longer than 12 months. There are several possible etiologies for dysphagia following anterior cervical spinal surgery. Neurologic damage may result from direct trauma or stretch trauma to the recurrent laryngeal nerve, superior laryngeal nerve, or glossopharyngeal nerve. Other common complications are summarized in Table 4–1.

For some patients, the problem can be addressed immediately and no long-term treatment is necessary. The assessment process may ultimately require long-term treatments, which are discussed later in the chapter. Table 4–2 summarizes the initial assessment process from which treatment may be initiated.

Surgical complications described for anterior cervical spinal surgery that may affect deglutition include edema, hematoma, infection, and denervation. The following are the most common:

1. Prevertebral soft tissue swelling and associated reduced epiglottic inversion may result in dysphagia following the surgery. The region of swelling on the posterior pharyngeal wall may approximate the epiglottis and prevent it from inverting. This causes a transient obstruction that traps the bolus, resulting in residue at the valleculae and pyriform sinuses.
2. Hypertonicity of the upper esophageal sphincter, as diagnosed by manometry, may result in dysphagia following anterior cervical spinal surgery. Hypertonicity of the upper esophageal sphincter may prevent passage of the bolus into the esophagus, resulting in pharyngeal residue.

Table 4–2. Etiologic factors for postoperative dysphagia after anterior cervical spinal surgery.*

Pain	Muscles of tongue, pharynx/larynx, (post ET)[†]
Edema	Tongue, pharynx, larynx, neck
Hematoma	Retropharyngeal space
Infection/abscess	Retropharyngeal space
Interruption of motor innervation	Ansa cervercalis RLN[‡] Pharyngeal plexus
Interruption of neuromuscular function	Anterior tongue Base of tongue
Injury to sensory innervation	SLN[§] Pharyngeal plexus
Mechanical factors	Perforation Bulky reconstruction plate Adhesions—posterior pharyngeal wall
Velopharyngeal incompetence	Palatal shortening Wound breakdown

*Adapted from Drennen et al.[1]
[†]ET = endotracheal tube
[‡]RLN = recurrent laryngeal nerve
[§]SLN = superior laryngeal nerve

3. Esophageal perforation is a rare but serious cause of dysphagia following this surgery (1 in 500). A perforation is often not recognized until the patient develops an abscess or a salivary fistula.

4. Bone graft size and positioning during this surgery must be optimal so there is not impingement or compression upon the posterior pharyngeal wall. Impingement or compression upon the pharyngeal wall may result in dysphagia.

5. Screw loosening was observed during Flexible Endoscopic Evaluation of Swallowing evaluation in one case, resulting in dysphagia following anterior cervical spinal surgery. The patient demonstrated symptoms of dysphagia 8 weeks postoperatively due to one of the screws used to fixate the spinal column loosening by 6 mm. The screw subsequently impinged upon the posterior pharyngeal wall, resulting in dysphagia, and required a repeat anterior surgery to remove it.

Table 4–3. Causes of abnormal oral phase swallowing after head and neck surgery.

Loss of Oral Sphincter

• Resection of lip
• Poor reapproximation of orbicularis oris
• Marginal mandibular and lingual nerve section

Dental Extractions

Floor of Mouth Resection

• Loss of glossoalveolar sulcus
• Tethering of anterior tongue

Tongue Resection

• Improper bolus preparation

Hard Palate Resection

• Loss of oronasal separation
• Nasal regurgitation

Mandibulectomy

• Loss of dentition
• Altered oral sphincter

HEAD AND NECK SURGERY

Head and neck surgery for neoplasms of the upper aerodigestive tract alters the anatomy, causes scarring, and may injure motor and sensory nerves. All these factors contribute to the presence of dysphagia in the postoperative period. In addition, many of these patients require reconstruction with **insensate tissue flaps** that can contribute to the discoordination of the swallowing mechanism or can even cause mechanical obstruction or diversion of the bolus into the airway. Head and neck surgery may result in disruption of any of the phases of swallowing.

Table 4–3 lists the causes of abnormal oral phase related to surgical resection of the lip, floor of the mouth, palate, or mandible. It should be kept in mind that there is no one-to-one relationship between surgery in one area and a specific swallowing problem. However, identification of the dysphagia after surgery must begin with the assessment of the site affected by the surgery.

Table 4–4. Dysphagia after oropharyngeal resection.

Soft Palate

- Loss of oropharyngeal suction pump
- Velopharyngeal insufficiency

Tonsil

- Altered mobility of lateral pharyngeal wall

Tongue Base

- Loss of laryngeal protection
- Loss of sensation
- Loss of laryngeal elevation

Table 4–5. Dysphagia after surgery of the hypopharynx.

Pyriform Sinus

- Scarring of lateral pharyngeal wall
- Injury to superior laryngeal nerve and loss of sensation

Posterior Pharyngeal Wall

- Adynamic insensate flap reconstruction
- Scarring and aspiration

Table 4–4 summarizes the common swallowing deficits after oropharyngeal resection. Table 4–5 presents the common problems after surgery in the hypopharynx.

Skull Base Surgery

Patients undergoing skull base surgery are at risk for injury to the lower cranial nerves, brainstem, brain parenchyma, and soft tissues of the upper aerodigestive tract, depending on tumor location. Injury to these vital structures can lead to dysfunction of speech, swallowing, and airway protection. In addition to the mentioned deficits, patients undergoing skull base surgery frequently need reconstruction with insensate soft tissue flaps, which may compound the deficit due to their bulk. After skull base surgery, patients frequently need enteral tubes, prolonged intubation and ventilation, and tracheostomies that further compound the swallowing deficits.

Table 4–6. Clinical manifestations of cranial nerve deficits.*

Dysfunctional Cranial Nerve	Clinical Manifestations
V	Impaired oral preparation and transport
VII	Drooling Impaired oral preparation Retention in gingivobuccal sulcus
IX and X	Delayed initiation of pharyngeal phase Nasal reflux Pharyngeal stasis and pooling Voice weakness or loss Aspiration
XII	Lack of awareness of food in mouth Impaired oral preparation Impaired oral transport

*Adapted from Fagan.[2]

Lower cranial neuropathies are common sequellae and/or complications of skull base surgery. A high vagal injury leads to ipsilateral laryngeal anesthesia and vocal cord paralysis. In addition, it also produces paralysis of the ipsilateral soft palate, loss of vagus-mediated relaxation of the cricopharyngeus muscle, and discoordination of the pharyngeal musculature. Therefore, a high vagal lesion, in addition to other cranial nerve or neurologic deficit, produces marked postoperative deglutition and airway morbidity. This can be compounded by injury to other lower cranial nerves such as IX or XII. Table 4–6 summarizes the clinical manifestations of cranial nerve deficits following head and neck and/or skull base surgery. Thus, surgical resection may not only affect anatomic structures but also the neurologic complications brought on by injured or damaged cranial nerves.

Floor of the Mouth

The floor of the mouth is considered a sulcus for saliva and food particles; however, when obliterated by surgery, the lack of this sulcus and the loss of mobility of the anterior tongue become major impairments during the preparation of the food bolus. All efforts should be made to protect the lingual nerve to preserve the sensation to the tongue.

Partial Glossectomy

Following partial glossectomy, near-normal swallowing and normal speech can be predicted if the patient can protrude the tongue past the sublabial crease. Small defects of the mobile tongue are repaired primarily. Large defects often cause the loss of tongue driving force and inability to propel the bolus posteriorly. The bolus is often improperly prepared, and, due to the lack of proper control, it may be presented to the oropharynx prematurely. Food and saliva will spill out of the oral cavity because of poor tongue mobility, a problem that is worsened if the oral sphincter has been altered.

Palate

Tumors of the hard palate that require partial or total maxillectomy affect both speech and swallowing. Resection results in loss of oronasal separation, which causes leakage of food into the nose and hypernasal speech with decreased intelligibility. Unilateral maxillectomy is usually best reconstructed with a dental prosthesis. Free microvascular flaps can be used to reconstruct large palatal defects in edentulous patients in whom a prosthesis would not be retained.

After soft palate resection, patients often have nasal regurgitation. The reconstruction options are limited, and defects in the soft palate are best managed by dental prostheses with extensions to close the nasopharyngeal isthmus.

Lips

The **orbicularis oris muscle** is crucial to the sphincteric function of the lips. This muscle is divided during lip-splitting procedures and must be carefully reapproximated during closure to restore function. The loss of lower lip sensation secondary to mental nerve injury makes sphincteric control difficult if not impossible.

Lip resection may hinder swallowing by creating difficulty in getting food into the mouth (microstomia). Motor denervation of the lower lip secondary to sacrifice of the marginal mandibular nerve often manifests itself as loss of sphincteric control, resulting in drooling.

Mandible

Mandibular defects of the midline arch cause problems with proper chewing, oral sphincter control, laryngeal suspension and elevation, and the driving force of the tongue.

Oropharynx

Resection of the lateral pharyngeal wall leads to decreased pharyngeal wall mobility, which alters oropharyngeal propulsion. The muscles of the base of the tongue assist in elevation of the larynx and are essential for the oropharyngeal propulsion pump and for adequate oral cavity—pharyngeal separation. Although partial resection is well tolerated, large defects often cause dysphagia. Reconstruction of large defects of the base of the tongue requires a sensate flap. Resection of even limited portions of the soft palate produces velopharyngeal insufficiency, alters the propulsion of the bolus, and can lead to poor oral-pharyngeal separation with early spillage of the bolus and aspiration before the pharyngeal swallow is initiated.

Hypopharyngeal Surgery

Resection of hypopharyngeal tumors arising on the posterior pharyngeal wall poses several problems for the rehabilitation of swallowing. Small defects (less than 2 cm) can be closed primarily, or the edges can be stitched to the prevertebral fascia. Reconstruction with a split thickness skin graft or radial forearm free flap provides a satisfactory closure of larger defects. However, neither one restores the motility of the posterior wall, and impairment of pharyngeal contraction leads to significant postoperative aspiration. Patients lose the normal gliding action of the hypopharynx on the vertebral fascia because of scarring of the posterior hypopharyngeal wall to the prevertebral fascia. Also, the reconstruction of this area, using grafts and flaps, is almost always devoid of sensation, which further weakens laryngeal protection.

Examination of patients who have undergone reconstruction using a radial forearm free flap or a split thickness skin graft may reveal scarring that has resulted in small, horizontal shelves along the posterior pharyngeal wall. These shelves hold and divert the food bolus anteriorly into the larynx and may retain secretions and ingested food. When enough food or saliva accumulates, the material is dumped anteriorly into the introitus of the larynx and can result in significant aspiration. Commercial products may be used to thicken liquids and foods so that sensation is increased and the transit time is increased, allowing additional time for laryngeal protection.

TRACHEOSTOMY

Between 43% and 83% of patients with tracheostomy tubes manifest signs of aspiration or aspiration pneumonia. Dysphagia is produced by

Table 4–7. Physiological changes following tracheostomy.

* Loss or change in airway resistance
* Inability to generate subglottic air pressure during the swallow
* Reduced ability to produce an effective cough
* Loss of sense of smell
* Loss of phonation
* Reduced mucosal sensitivity
* Reduced true vocal fold closure and coordination
* Disruption of the respiration/swallowing cycle
* Foreign body effect
* Reduced laryngeal elevation during deglutition

the physiological changes associated with opening the trachea to atmospheric pressure, not merely the presence of the tube in the neck. Table 4–7 summarizes the most common physiological changes following tracheostomy.

Airway Pressure Changes

A major factor contributing to aspiration is that a tracheostomy results in a reduction in **airway resistance.** Expiratory resistance during respiration is provided by the vocal folds, with a constant resistance of about 8 to 10 cm/H_2O/liter/sec. This "braking" helps maintain lung inflation through physiological prolongation of the expiratory phase. Pressure measurements during swallowing with a tracheostomy are similar to that with an occluded airway and are lost with an open airway. This pressure is present in the trachea following glottic closure during swallowing, and peaks at about 8 to 10 cm/H_2O. Subglottic air pressure seems to be critical to swallow function. Its restoration reverses, at least in part, the disordered swallowing function that accompanies tracheostomy.

Expiratory Speaking Valves

Decannulation or even tube occlusion will enhance swallowing function in a patient with a tracheostomy. However, this is not feasible in all patients. An alternative strategy is to place an **expiratory speaking**

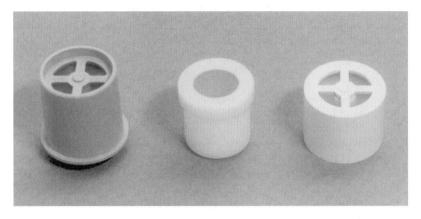

Figure 4–1. Three speaking valves: Passy-Muir valve for ventilators (left), Montgomery valve (center), and Passy-Muir valve (right). From Gross RD, Eibling DE. Tracheostomy/endotracheal intubation. Chapter 20. In: Carrau RL, Murry T, eds. *Comprehensive Management of Swallowing Disorders.* San Diego, Calif: Singular Publishing Group; 1999:137.

valve on the open tracheostomy tube, which restores subglottic air pressure during swallowing (Figure 4–1). The beneficial effect of a valve strengthens the fact that subglottic air pressure is a critical factor in swallowing efficiency, probably through restoring proprioceptive cues.

Laryngeal Elevation

The vertical motion of the larynx is dependent on the function of the suprahyoid musculature and results in shortening of the pharynx and simultaneous active opening of the cricopharyngeal sphincter. Laryngeal elevation is reduced following tracheostomy and probably plays a significant role in the dysphagia associated with the procedure.

Glottic Closure

Lung protection is provided by cessation of respiration and the maintenance of glottic closure. In the typical individual, swallowing is timed to occur during expiration. This relationship is lost in patients with severe respiratory disease and is also lost or severely altered in the presence of a tracheostomy.

Glottic closure during swallowing is an extremely basic reflex that is mediated by the superior laryngeal nerve (uncrossed) and requires

18 to 40 milliseconds. This rapid response suggests that the reflex arc is located in the lower brainstem and does not require input from higher centers. The laryngeal surface of the epiglottis and the other supraglottic structures are richly endowed with receptors, including water receptors. Interruption of sensory input by the superior laryngeal nerve or high vagal nerve interruption limits the glottic closure reflex and contributes to aspiration. Disruption of the integrity of the subglottic airway—thus allowing the building of subglottic pressure—by the presence of a tracheostomy also blunts or eliminates the glottic closure reflex.

Pharyngeal Transit

Bolus transit from the tongue base to the esophagus requires less than a second in the typical individual. Prolongation of bolus transit time, as well as disruption of the glottic closure, results in food or liquid being in the pharynx while the glottis is open and, thus, places the individual at risk for aspiration. It has been demonstrated that this transit time can be prolonged in the presence of a tracheostomy and that this effect is reversible. Restricted range of motion of pharyngeal structures such as may be associated with the tethering of the larynx by the presence of a tracheostomy tube is likely to also affect transit time.

ZENKER'S DIVERTICULUM

Zenker's diverticulum is a **pulsion diverticulum** that forms above the cricopharyngeal sphincter muscle through an area of lesser muscle strength termed **Killian's triangle.** The diverticulum is created by failure of the upper esophageal sphincter to open before the peristaltic wave and by failure of active opening of the cricopharyngeal muscle through weakness of the laryngeal elevators.

As surgery is the only time-proven therapeutic option for Zenker's diverticulum, the decision to operate is driven by the degree of the patient's symptoms. Typical symptoms are summarized in Table 4–8. These include regurgitation of partially digested food, potentially foul smelling and resulting in halitosis; dysphagia; coughing and choking on swallowing; inanition and weight loss; esophageal obstruction; and recurrent aspiration pneumonia.

Symptomatic patients who desire excision and can tolerate anesthesia are candidates for excision. The indications and contraindications are shown in Table 4–9. Surgical treatment options are many and include a range of options from open cricopharyngeal myotomy for

Table 4–8. Symptoms of Zenker's diverticulum.*

Symptom	Patients (%)
Dysphagia	48 (100)
Aspiration	20 (42)
Postdeglutitive cough	17 (35)
Regurgitation	14 (29)
Noisy swallowing	13 (27)
Weight loss (>10 lbs)	13 (27)
Recumbent cough	10 (21)
Sore throat	8 (17)
Unable to swallow	8 (17)
Halitosis	2 (4)

*Adapted from Schmidt and Zuckerbraun.[3]

Table 4–9. Zenker's diverticulum: surgical indications and contraindications.*

Indications	Contraindications
• Coughing and choking on swallowing • Recurrent aspiration pneumonia • Regurgitation/halitosis • Inanition/weight loss • Dysphagia • Esophageal obstruction	• Inability to withstand general anesthesia • Carcinoma of the esophagus • Untreated severe GERD (relative)

*Adapted from Goldberg and Eibling.[4]

small diverticula to myotomy with excision of the sack. Small diverticula can be observed if symptoms are tolerated by the patient.

Absolute contraindications to surgery include inability to tolerate general anesthesia (a significant consideration in the elderly population in which Zenker's diverticula are found) and carcinoma of the esophagus (which has been rarely reported within the actual diverticular pouch). The presence of untreated severe gastroesophageal reflux disease (GERD) is a relative contraindication.

External approaches to Zenker's diverticula have been used with considerable success since the beginning of the twentieth century. Cricopharyngeal myotomy is performed in conjunction with external approaches, typically prior to the removal, pexy, or imbrication of the diverticulum. Endoscopic approaches for the management of Zenker's diverticula have been performed successfully for the last 40 years. The mucosa and the cricopharyngeus muscle, which make up the party wall between the diverticular pouch and the esophagus, are divided. Prolonged follow-up of the patient is recommended, though no specific guidelines for reevaluation have been established. Yearly follow-up appears to be a logical interval.

REFERENCES

1. Drennen K, Welch W, Carrau RL. In: Carrau RL, Murry T, eds. *Comprehensive Management of Swallowing Disorders*. San Diego, Calif: Singular Publishing Group; 1999:166, 169.
2. Fagan J. In: Carrau RL, Murry T, eds. *Comprehensive Management of Swallowing Disorders*. San Diego, Calif: Singular Publishing Group; 1999:212.
3. Schmidt PJ, Zuckerbraun L. Treatment of Zenker's diverticula by cricopharyngeal myotomy under local anesthesia. *Am Surg.* 1992; 58:710–716.
4. Goldberg AN, Eibling DE. Pathophysiology of Zenker's diverticulum. In: Carrau RL, Murry T, eds. *Comprehensive Management of Swallowing Disorders*. San Diego, Calif: Singular Publishing Group; 1999:195–198.

5

Evaluation of Dysphagia

INTRODUCTION

The evaluation of swallowing encompasses the case history, the clinical or bedside swallow examination and the instrumental examination. In many assessment protocols, the case history and bedside swallow evaluation are combined. Each aspect of the swallow evaluation is designed to address the issues of (1) swallow safety, (2) nutritional status, (3) continuation or possible modification of present diet, and (4) need and appropriateness for additional instrumental tests.

THE BEDSIDE SWALLOW EVALUATION

The clinician should be prepared to find answers to the following questions as a result of conducting a thorough case history and bedside swallow evaluation: (1) What is the anatomic and functional status of the oral mechanism? (2) Is there a risk of aspiration given the present nutritional status and diet? (3) Should the patient be referred for further evaluation? (4) Is the patient cognitively capable of participating in instrumental testing and rehabilitation? (5) What changes in the treatment plan should be anticipated or planned given the diagnosis?

With these questions in mind, the clinician must understand that the bedside swallow evaluation has significant limitations since it does not include an anatomic examination of the pharynx and larynx. Moreover, depending on the status of the patient (e.g., severe impairment from stroke or extensive trauma), a complete bedside swallow evaluation is sometimes not possible. Despite the limitations of this evaluation, for patients with these problems, a limited bedside swallow evaluation may be the only basis for the decision to begin or suspend oral feeding or to recommend a **nasogastric** (NG) or **percutaneous endoscopic gastrostomy** (PEG) feeding tube. Thus, the bedside swallow evaluation, with its case history component, is an extremely important and valuable tool in the diagnostic process despite its caveats.[1]

Case History

Chief Complaint. Table 5–1 summarizes the critical components of the case history. Prior to any assessment of the patient, the clinician should identify the chief complaint or define the current status of the patient. The detailed history should account for the current physical status, including any recent surgeries or conditions from previous surgeries that may contribute to the dysphagia. The onset of the dysphagia should be documented and related to events such as surgery, neurologic changes, medicines, or trauma (physical or emotional). Based on the patient's input, family input, or medical records, the severity of the problem should be determined. Time since oral food intake, anatomic changes to the swallowing mechanism, neurologic status, and degree of alertness help to make those determinations.

Clinical findings noted in the medical records should be considered. Common clinical findings that are associated with dysphagia

Table 5–1. Critical components of the clinical case history.*

- Identify the chief complaint or define the current status
- Onset, progression
- Time elapsed from initiation of swallow to symptoms
- Associated symptoms
- Present and past
  Illnesses
  Surgery
  Trauma
- Medications
- Trauma
- Social history/habits
- Family history
- Review of systems

*Adapted from Carrau.[2]

and/or aspiration are shown in Table 5–2. Note that even when the majority of these symptoms are absent, swallow safety may still be an important issue. Both Table 5–1 and Table 5–2 illustrate that the importance of observing the patient, reviewing the case history, and acquiring information from caregivers are important aspects of the bedside swallow evaluation.

Silent Aspiration

The clinician must always be aware of the possibility of **silent aspiration.** This is the penetration of food, liquid, or saliva to the subglottic area without the elicitation of a cough. It has been estimated that silent aspiration may be as high as 40% in patients with dysphagia, and it is not generally identifiable during the bedside swallow evaluation.

The Oropharyngeal Examination

The **oropharyngeal examination** should include an assessment of lip closure, tongue strength, and mobility; facial symmetry; and the voice strength and volitional cough strength. Table 5–3, modified from Daniels et al,[4] provides a comprehensive, orderly approach to the

Table 5–2. Common clinical findings in dysphagic patients.*

- Coughing/choking—swallowing food, liquid, or own saliva
- Frequent throat clearing—with or without a productive cough
- Multiple swallow pattern
- Wet vocal quality
- Edentulous
- Drooling
- Increased oral or pharyngeal secretions
- Cyanosis
- Shortness of breath
- Weight loss
- Bronchorrhea
- Increased time to consume meal
- Spiking fever
- Pulmonary infiltrate
- Resistance to eating or drinking
- Food sticking in mouth
- Changes in taste
- Difficulty in managing foods of specific textures or sensation
- Aberrant behavioral patterns when food is presented

*Adapted from Simonian and Goldberg.[3]

Table 5–3. The oropharyngeal examination for the bedside swallow evaluation.*

Name _____   Date _____
Diagnosis _____

Mandible (CN V)
　Symmetry on Extension _____   Strength _____

Lips (CN VII)
　Symmetry: Rest _____   Retraction _____ Protrusion _____
　Strength _____
　Nonspeech Coordination: Repetitive Movement _____ Alternating Movement ____
　Speech Coordination: Repetitive (/p,w/) _____ Alternating (/p–w/)

Tongue (CN XII)
　Symmetry: Rest _____ Protrusion _____ Lateralization _____
　Elevation **Yes/No**　　　　　　Lateralization **Yes/No**　　Fasciculations
Yes/No
　Strength _____   _____
　Nonspeech Coordination: Repetitive Movement _____ Alternating Movement _____
　Speech Coordination: Repetitive (/t,k/) _____ Alternating (/t–k/) _____
　Alternating Movement (/p^t^k^/) _____
　Multisyllabic Word Repetition (tip top, baseball player, several, caterpillar, emphasize)
　_____
　Conversation: (speech, voice, coordination characteristics) _____
　Laryngeal Function: Isolated Movement (/i–i–i/ on one breath) _____
　Alternating Movement (/u–i/) _____
　Buccofacial Apraxia; "Blow out the candle" _____ "Lick an ice cream cone" _____
　"Lick milk off your top lip" _____ "Sip through a straw" _____ "Kiss a baby" _____

Velum (CN IX, X, XI)
　Symmetry: Rest _____   Elevation _____
　Coordination: Repetitive Movement (/a/) _____
　Appearance of Hard Palate _____
　Dentition _____

Reflexes (CN IX, X, XI)
　Gag (Abnormal: **Yes/No**) _____
　Swallow (Cough: **Yes/No**) _____
　　(Voice Change: **Yes/No**) _____

Additional Information
　c/o Facial Numbness or Tingling: **Yes/No**　Light Touch _____
　Dysphonia: **Yes/No** (mild, moderate, severe) _____
　Dysarthria: **Yes/No** (mild, moderate, severe) _____
　Breath Support _____
　Resonance _____
　Volitional Cough (Abnormal: **Yes/No**)

_____   _____
　Clinician　　　　　　　　　　　Date

*Adapted with permission from Daniels et al.[4]

oropharyngeal examination. Clinicians, even those with extensive experience in oral examination, may profit from this structure because of its approach to assessing muscular function related to the cranial nerves most important for swallowing.

Prior to the oropharyngeal examination, the clinician should have a general knowledge of the patient characteristics that may interfere with parts of the examination. These include

1. Airway
2. Cognition/alertness/endurance
3. Ability to follow instructions
4. Body tone/size/posture/positioning
5. Self-feeding potential

Oral Phase Examination. The oral examination should include assessment of the range of motion, strength, and sensory function of all oral structures. Prominent atrophy and fasciculation of the tongue should raise the possibility of amyotrophic lateral sclerosis (ALS). The examination should include the following:

1. Reflexes and responses
   - The gag reflex includes a head and jaw extension, rhythmical tongue protrusions, and pharyngeal contractions in response to stimulation at the posterior part of the oral cavity. Recent literature suggests that the gag reflex may not be important for normal swallowing to occur.
   - The bite reflex is clamping of the teeth or up and down movement of the jaw in response to stimulation of the gum, molar, or other dental surfaces.
   - The transverse tongue response is a lateral movement in response to tactile stimulation at the lateral border.
2. Sensation: Assess by light touch of lips and tongue.
3. Structural anatomy: Look for abnormalities of lips and oral cavity.
4. Movement
   - Jaw: Ability to open and close the jaw.
   - Lips: Labial closure at rest and during swallowing.
   - Tongue: Anterior lingual movement may be assessed by having the patient extend, lateralize, elevate, and depress the tip, and by having the patient sweep the tongue from front to back along the roof of the mouth.
   - Velum: Movement of the velum, or soft palate, may be assessed by having the patient open the mouth and then observing palatal movement during production of a sustained /a/ sound.
5. Secretions: Note location and amount.

6. Articulation: Screen with sentences or words containing tongue tip and posterior tongue consonants.
7. Resonance: Note presence of hypernasal quality.

Pharyngeal and Laryngeal Evaluation. The pharyngeal and laryngeal examination should include asessment of the following:

1. Vocal quality/changes
2. Pitch control/range
3. Breathing
4. Volitional cough/throat clearing
5. Saliva swallow: Laryngeal management
6. Laryngeal elevation

Clinical Swallow Evaluation

The final portion of the bedside swallow evaluation consists of trial swallows of water. The clinician should be consistent in the amount of water to be swallowed. The majority of reports suggest that beginning with a 5-ml bolus is appropriate.[5] Depending on the results, one can advance to 10-ml and 20-ml boluses. **Laryngeal elevation,** identified by palpation of the thyroid prominence, should be monitored for each swallow. After each swallow, the patient is asked to sustain the /a/ vowel for a few seconds or count from 1 to 5 to determine if there is wet hoarseness or other change in voice quality. Daniels and her associates[4] suggest that wet hoarseness and a weak cough are two signs of increased risk for aspiration.

The physical examination should include a basic head and neck and neurologic examination with assessment of gait, balance, and sensory and motor function of the extremities; deep tendon reflexes; and full assessment of the cranial nerves outlined in Table 5–4. This may be done by a speech language pathologist, neurologist, or otolaryngologist; or they may do it as a team.

Laryngeal Examination

For those patients with a weak or breathy voice, a consultation with an otolaryngologist is recommended. The otolaryngologist may perform an examination of the larynx and vocal folds using a **flexible endoscope.**

During the flexible laryngoscopy, the anatomy of the pharynx and larynx should be observed during quiet and forced respiration, coughing, speaking, and swallowing. Attention is also given to the motion of the base of the tongue, pharyngeal walls, arytenoids, and

Table 5–4. Bedside clinical evaluation: physical examination.*

Oral

- Oral continence
  Lip pursing
  "Trumpeter" maneuvers
  Drooling
- Tongue range of motion
  Extends beyond lower lip
  Approximates to gingivobuccal area
  Can push against tongue blade
- Tongue sensation

Oropharynx

- Motion of soft palate
- Sensation
  Tongue blade/swab
  Cold laryngeal mirror
  Gag reflex
  Swallow reflex

Flexible Laryngoscopy

- Anatomy of base of tongue, vallecula, hypopharynx, endolarynx
- Pooling of secretions
- Penetration/aspiration of secretions
- Motion (symmetry, range) of base of tongue, arytenoid, epiglottis, false vocal cords, true vocal cords (fixation vs. paralysis)
- Velopharyngeal closure
  Lateral walls
  Passavant's ridge
  Velum

Neck

- Laryngeal elevation
- Adenopathy
- Thyroid
- Other masses

Neurological

- Cranial nerves
- Gait/balance
- Motor function/fine skills
- Deep tendon reflexes

*Adapted from Carrau.[2]

other endolaryngeal structures. Symmetry, coordination, and range of movement between the two sides of the upper aerodigestive tract are also noted. Pooling of secretions or food residue in the vallecula or piriform sinuses is noted. The laryngeal closure reflex can be tested by gentle touch of the epiglottis or aryepiglottic folds with the tip of the endoscope. This maneuver requires some experience and should be as gentle as possible to avoid eliciting a gag reflex or laryngospasm. A more detailed assessment of sensation is presented later in this chapter. The neck is examined for swelling or masses. Observation of the thyroid movement and prominence upon swallowing reflects laryngeal evaluation.

OPTIMAL PROTOCOLS

Other options in place of the bedside swallow evaluation have been proposed by DePippo et al.[6] They found that cough or voice change during or directly after drinking 3 oz of water was a sensitive and valid screening tool for aspiration following a stroke. It should be remembered that the clinical swallow assessment with water should be tried only after the findings from the patient history and oropharyngeal examination are taken into account. Patients unable to tolerate their secretions, who have limited attention such as those shortly after a severe stroke, or who resist for some other reason may not be candidates for the clinical water swallow test.

Dysphagia Screening

Prior to a formal bedside swallow evaluation and, in some settings, in place of the complete bedside swallow evaluation, the use of a dysphagia screening test may be appropriate. This is usually done by a speech and language pathologist but may also be done by a nurse trained in the procedure. Two such screening tests are the Burke Dysphagia Screening Test (BDST)[7] and the screening test proposed by Odderson and McKenna.[8] The BDST consists of a seven-item test. Presence of one or more of the items in the test results in failure and referral for a complete bedside swallow evaluation. The screening items are (1) bilateral stroke, (2) brainstem stroke, (3) history of pneumonia in the acute stroke phase, (4) cough during the 3-oz water swallow or associated with feeding, (5) failure to consume one half of meals, (6) prolonged time required for feeding (greater than 30 minutes and the time not caused by physical limitations), and (7) non-oral feeding program in progress. This screening procedure, as well as that proposed by Odderson and McKenna, was given to stroke patients and found to be highly valuable in identifying patients at risk for swallowing problems.

Although the majority of bedside swallow evaluation reports focus on stroke patients, there are reports that relate findings from the clinical bedside assessment of swallowing to other patient groups. In general, these findings suggest that for surgical patients, the larger the surgical excision, the more likely the patient will exhibit more extensive and a longer course of dysphagia. Patients in these categories require more extensive evaluation and treatments.

Dye Test

The **dye test,** also known as the **blue dye test,** may be used to determine the presence of aspiration in a tracheostomized patient. A few drops of methylene blue or vegetable coloring are placed in the mouth, the tracheostomy cuff is deflated, and the tracheostomy tube is deep suctioned for secretions that may have been resting on or above the level of the cuff. The patient's tracheostomy tube is deep suctioned again, this time looking for evidence of dyed material in the airway. The blue dye test, however, may not detect trace amounts of aspirated materials. Recent research suggests that trace aspiration and delayed aspiration may not be reliably identified using this procedure. Alternatively, a Dextrostix® may be used to detect the presence of glucose (i.e., food) in the tracheal secretions.

Auscultation: Chest and Cervical

Auscultation of the chest and cervical airway is done by placing a stethoscope over various parts of the airway. Placing the stethoscope gently on the lateral aspect of the larynx and listening to the airflow during normal breathing, swallowing, and speech provide the listener with indirect evidence of penetration and/or aspiration.

Once the clinical evaluation is completed, the clinician will be able to establish a reasonable differential diagnosis (Table 5–5) and determine which other tests are needed. Table 5–6 summarizes the more commonly used tests used to study dysphagia, along with their application and utility.

Table 5–5. Differential diagnosis.*

Type	Possible Etiology
Congenital	Dysphagia lusoria Tracheoesophageal fistula Laryngeal clefts Other foregut abnormalities
Inflammatory	GERD
Infections	Lyme disease Neuropathies/encephalitis Chagas' disease
Trauma	CNS Upper aerodigestive tract Surgical injury
Endocrine	Goiter Hypothyroid Diabetic neuropathy
Neoplasia	Upper aerodigestive tract Thyroid Central nervous system

Systemic	Autoimmune
	  Dermatomyositis
	  Scleroderma
	  Sjögren's
	Amyloidosis
	Sarcoidosis

Iatrogenic	Surgery Chemotherapy Other medications Radiation

*Adapted from Carrau.[2]

Table 5–6. Functional evaluation of swallowing: tests most commonly used and their usefulness for identifying various aspects of swallowing disorders.

	Defines Anatomy	Detects Aspiration	Quantifies Aspiration	Detects Etiology	Availability	Cost*
Bedside Evaluation	–	+/–†	–	+/–	++	1
MBS	+	++	+	+	+	3
FEES	++	+	–	+	++	2
Ultrasound	+/–	–	–	–	+/–	4
Scintigraphy	–	++	++	–	+/–	6
Manometry	–	+/‡	–	+	+	5

Key: + Useful for evaluating
++ Highly desirable to make diagnosis
– Does not apply
*Order from least to most expensive
†Can detect actual aspiration in patients with tracheostomies
‡Quantifies Reflux

INSTRUMENTAL TESTS OF SWALLOW FUNCTION

Modified Barium Swallow

Test Procedure. The **modified barium swallow** is also called a video-fluorographic swallowing study. The term "cookie swallow" has been used in the past, but it is misleading and does not adequately describe the procedure. The test is more comprehensive than swallowing a cookie and involves the use of technical instrumentation and expertise to assess the results. The modified barium swallow is a multidisciplinary evaluation of the swallowing mechanism involving collaboration between a radiologist and a speech and language pathologist (SLP).[5] The modified barium swallow is a dynamic assessment of the oral, pharyngeal, and esophageal phases of swallowing by means of videofluoroscopy. This examination provides a comprehensive instrumental assessment of swallowing and follows the bedside swallow evaluation when dysphagia risk factors outlined in the previous section are identified. The decision to recommend a modified barium swallow test is often based on the findings of the clinical bedside evaluation. The test requires a fluoroscopic unit, video recorder, a chair suitable to stabilize the patient, and various food and liquids that will be coated or mixed with barium.

Under **fluoroscopic observation,** controlled by the radiologist, the patient ingests barium-coated boluses or liquid barium of varying consistencies, which is offered at the discretion of the speech and language pathologist. The modified barium swallow usually starts with a thin liquid barium preparation, unless there is evidence of choking on liquids. Thickened barium liquid, pudding, and solids (usually pieces of cookie or a marshmallow coated with barium) are also commonly used in this test. These consistencies are chosen to approximate the consistencies of food that a patient is likely to encounter in his or her daily diet. Some clinicians use other preparations, such as deviled chicken and beef stew, to test the patient's ability to handle different consistencies of food.

Frontal and lateral x-ray views are obtained with the fluoroscope in a fixed position during the modified barium swallow with the patient standing or sitting. The procedure is purely dynamic; the study is recorded on videotape. It can be used immediately to test for various consistencies, postures in swallowing, or techniques to manage the bolus. With this videotaped information, the goals can be set and the treatment is defined.

Modified Barium Swallow Test Observations. The modified barium swallow concentrates on the oral, oropharyngeal, and hypopharyngeal phases of deglutition, although it is also useful to perform a brief evaluation of the esophagus. This dynamic study evaluates formation of the bolus in the mouth, tongue motion, coordination, timing and completeness of swallowing, movement of the epiglottis, elevation of the larynx, and cricopharyngeal contraction. Because of the potential danger of exposure to radiation, the clinician must select consistencies wisely to limit radiation exposure.

The modified barium swallow is an excellent test for evaluating the oral and pharyngeal phase of swallowing. Pathology that may explain the presence of dysphagia, such as abnormal movements of the tongue in forming the bolus and initiating deglutition, residual barium that pools in the valleculae or piriform sinuses, and aspiration of barium into the airway, can be identified. Because the entire fluoroscopic study is recorded on videotape, the study can provide a highly detailed analysis of the coordination and timing of swallowing. The modified barium swallow may also include testing with compensatory and swallowing maneuvers, such as the chin tuck, supraglottic swallow, or Mendelsohn maneuver, to name just a few. These postures and maneuvers are discussed in Chapter 6.

Entry of barium into the airway may be the most important observation that the team performing the modified barium swallow can

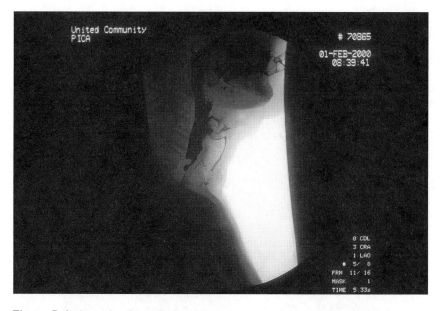

Figure 5–1. Lateral radiograph showing contrast material in esophagus and airway.

make. The clearest and most clinically useful solution to the problem of terminology to describe barium in the airway is to state the location of the barium that extends lowest into the airway. This may be as subtle as coating of the laryngeal surface of the epiglottis (i.e., penetration) or as obvious as gross aspiration of barium into the lower tracheo-bronchial tree (Figure 5–1). The location and extent of aspiration should be defined clearly. Rosenbek and his colleagues[9] proposed an eight-step scale to evaluate the degree of penetration and aspiration seen on the modified barium swallow. The eight-step scale may be quite useful to monitor changes in a patient's ability to control aspiration and advance to another eating level. Material

1. does not enter airway
2. remains above folds/ejected from airway
3. remains above folds/not ejected from airway
4. contacts folds/ejected from airway
5. contacts folds/not ejected from airway
6. passes below folds/ejected into larynx or out of airway
7. passes below folds/not ejected despite effort
8. passes below folds/no spontaneous effort to eject

While these steps may not be exact intervals, they do describe decreasing swallow safety from no penetration to aspiration. As with the "traditional" barium swallow, nasopharyngeal reflux of barium should also be documented during the modified barium swallow (Figure 5–2).

The Modified Barium Swallow and Causes of Aspiration. The modified barium swallow can often provide information as to the cause of aspiration, but it does not necessarily predict aspiration. Abnormal motion of the epiglottis, diminished contractions of the pharyngeal constrictor muscles, and abnormal laryngeal "rise" can all be identified on the

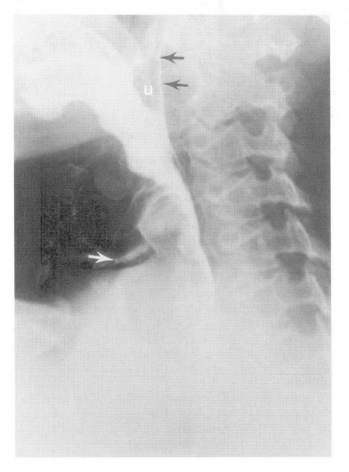

Figure 5–2. Nasopharyngeal reflux and tracheal aspiration. Lateral view from a barium swallow shows barium (*black arrows*) extending above the uvula (*u*) and soft palate. This is nasopharyngeal reflux. There is also barium in the trachea (*white arrow*), indicating that the patient aspirated. From Carrau RL, Murry T, eds. *Comprehensive Management of Swallowing Disorders.* San Diego, Calif: Singular Publishing Group; 1999:68.

modified barium swallow. Silent aspiration is aspiration into the tracheobronchial tree that fails to elicit a normal cough response to clear the barium. Silent aspiration offers evidence of an underlying neurologic dysfunction related to the loss or diminution of sensation. Silent aspiration may remain undetected on clinical (bedside) swallow examination but is readily apparent from the fluoroscopic record of the modified barium swallow.

If barium enters the airway, the effectiveness of **airway protective maneuvers** and varying the consistency of the barium bolus can be assessed directly by viewing under fluoroscopy. Fluoroscopic examination has been shown to be far more sensitive for detecting even small amounts of aspirated material than a bedside swallowing study.

Fiberoptic Endoscopic Evaluation of Swallowing

The Procedure. The **Fiberoptic Endoscopic Evaluation of Swallowing** assessment was first described by Langmore et al.[10] The assessment of swallowing using this technique requires the passage of a **fiberoptic laryngoscope** into the nares, over the velum to a position above the epiglottis (Figure 5–3 A and B). The fiberoptic endoscopic evaluation of swallowing is an assessment of swallowing using a flexible nasoendoscope to evaluate the swallow before and after the pharyngeal swallow.

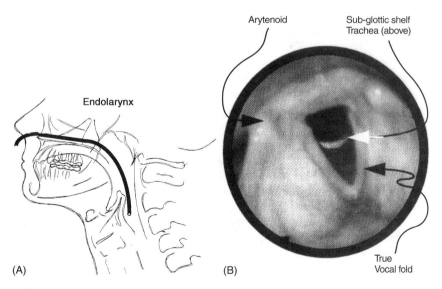

Figure 5–3. Fiberoptic endoscopic evaluation of swallowing diagram. From Perlman A, Schulze-Delrieu K. *Deglutition and Its Disorders: Anatomy, Physiology, Clinical Diagnosis, and Management.* San Diego, Calif: Singular Publishing Group; 1999:209.

Specific amounts of liquids and food consistencies treated with food dye are viewed as they pass the pharynx and larynx. During the time of airway closure, the swallow cannot be visualized, as the pharyngeal walls contract over the bolus, collapsing the lumen over the endoscope (**whiteout phase**). Monitoring of the bolus is only possible before and after the pharyngeal swallow. However, the bolus can be monitored as it enters into view from the oral cavity to the pharynx. A video camera and recorder coupled to the endoscope provide a permanent record of the examination for later review by clinicians and patient and serve as a baseline to monitor the patient's progress. This test is often performed by an otolaryngologist and speech and language pathologist. In selected cases, fiberoptic endoscopic evaluation of swallowing can provide a patient with visual feedback that may aid the rehabilitation process.

The Examination. Before liquid or food is offered to the patient, the endoscope is placed and the examiner notes the anatomic structures and observes the functions of the velum palatinum, epiglottis, and larynx, using sustained phonation or repeating "Coca Cola." Trial "dry" swallows to observe laryngeal elevation are prompted, and phonation to observe vocal fold closure is elicited. The amount of retained secretions present in the vallecula and hypopharynx is also noted. Figure 5–4 shows a photograph with retained secretions. Pharyngeal and laryngeal functions should be documented with different bolus consistencies and amounts, along with various positional changes of the head. The supraglottic swallow and chin tuck strategies may also be used to determine appropriate methods for protecting the airway and for improving clearance of the retained secretions in the piriform sinuses.

The speed of the pharyngeal swallow, premature flow of food or liquid into the pharyngeal and laryngeal areas, and residual amounts of the bolus can all be seen during this examination. The endoscope may remain in place for long periods to monitor the residual bolus and examine anatomic structures. Swallowing, using compensatory strategies and changes in neck position, is easily accomplished while the endoscope is in place.

The fiberoptic endoscopic evaluation of swallowing examination is more sensitive than the modified barium swallow in detecting subtle abnormalities of the palate, pharynx, and larynx, thus providing better anatomic information than the modified barium swallow. The fiberoptic endoscopic evaluation of swallowing, however, does not completely assess the oral phase and does not evaluate aspiration during the swallow. This assessment may not be indicated for patients

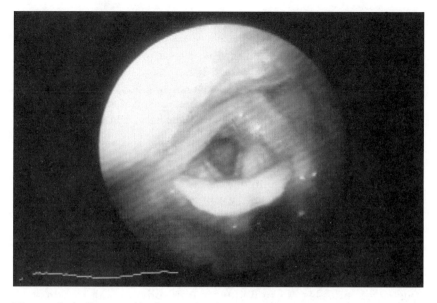

Figure 5–4. Photographic image showing retained secretions in the vallecula.

with extreme movement disorders, those who cannot tolerate the endoscopes, or those who have a history of severe bronchospasm or laryngospasm.

Fiberoptic Endoscopic Evaluation of Swallowing with Sensory Testing

This procedure employs the standard fiberoptic endoscopic testing with the addition of **sensory testing** of the supraglottic mucosa to determine the presence of a sensory dysfunction in dysphagic patients. To perform the test, an air pulse generator is used to send a pulse of air through a port in a specially designed flexible nasopharyngoscope. Air pulses can be delivered to the supraglottic larynx and pharynx areas. Using a calibrated puff of air, sensory thresholds can then be determined using one of the psychophysical testing methods. The twitch response of the mucosa suggests the sensory awareness of the stimulus. The fiberoptic endoscopic evaluation of swallowing with sensory testing provides an accurate indication of the sensory function or dysfunction of the aryepiglottic space, which in turn reflects the degree of awareness of bolus in the oropharynx and the need to protect the airway.

Manometry

Esophageal manometry provides a qualitative as well as a quantitative assessment of esophageal motility, pressures, and coordination. Manometry is used in the evaluation of **esophageal motility disorders,** including achalasia and diffuse esophageal spasm. It is also important in the identification of motor abnormalities associated with other systemic diseases such as scleroderma, diabetes mellitus, and chronic intestinal pseudo-obstruction.

Pharyngeal manometry can be performed in conjunction with esophageal motility studies. Normally, the response of the oropharynx to swallowing has two components. The first is compression of the catheter against the pharyngeal wall by the tongue, which results in a high, sharp-peaked amplitude pressure wave. This is followed by a low-amplitude, long-duration wave, which reflects the initiation of pharyngeal peristalsis. A rapid, high-amplitude pressure upstroke ending in a single, sharp peak, followed by a rapid return to baseline, is produced by the contraction of the middle and inferior pharyngeal constrictor muscles to provide the mid-pharyngeal response to swallowing.

The pharynx is not radially symmetrical, and, therefore, the measurements obtained during standard manometry vary with the catheter placement. Nonetheless, measurements of intrabolus pressures during the pharyngeal phase of swallowing may predict which patients will respond to a surgical myotomy.

A **polyvinyl catheter,** a thin tube about 35 cm long made of a flexible polyvinyl material and constructed with multiple pressure sensors, is passed transnasally, and the patient is instructed to perform a series of wet and dry swallows (Figure 5–5). Lower esophageal sphincter pressure is measured at baseline and in response to a swallow. Figure 5–6 shows a catheter reading from the testing. Lower esophageal sphincter pressure is measured as a step up in pressure from the gastric baseline referenced as atmospheric. Complete lower esophageal sphincter relaxation with a swallow is demonstrated by a decrease in pressure to gastric baseline for approximately 6 seconds. Basal upper esophageal sphincter pressures can be identified as a rise in pressure above the esophageal baseline. Due to the asymmetry of the upper esophageal sphincter, this is normally 50 to 100 mm Hg depending on the direction of the pressure sensor (i.e. whether lateral or anterior/posterior). Evaluation of upper esophageal sphincter relaxation and correlation of sphincter relaxation with pharyngeal contraction is obtained by instructing the patient to perform a series of wet swallows.

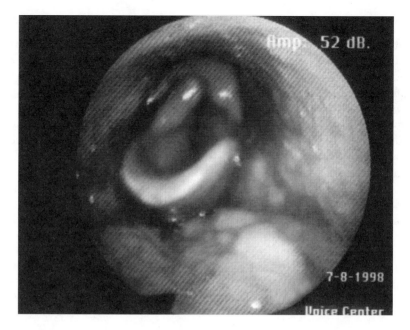

Figure 5–5. Fiberoptic endoscopic evaluation of swallowing procedure. View of larynx following swallow of liquid by a 58-year-old male with bilateral vocal fold paresis and atrophy. Note the presence of liquid on the right vocal fold and a drop of liquid between the vocal folds, anteriorly.

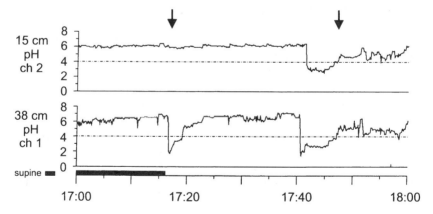

Figure 5–6. One hour of a 24-hour ambulatory pH recording from the distal and proximal esophagus shows two episodes of reflux. Each reflux episode is labeled with an arrow. In the second reflux episode, acid reflux in the distal esophagus reaches the proximal esophagus or higher. Adapted from Padda S, Young MA. Chapter 13. In: Carrau RL, Murry T, eds. *Comprehensive Management of Swallowing Disorders.* San Diego, Calif: Singular Publishing Group; 1999:85.

Ultrasound

Ultrasound uses high frequency sounds (>2 MHz) from a transducer held or fixed in contact with skin to obtain a dynamic image of soft tissues. As ultrasound does not penetrate bone, its use is limited to the soft tissues of the oral cavity and parts of the oropharynx. Ultrasound is completely noninvasive and does not use ionizing radiation; therefore, repeated studies can be done without risk. It is highly efficient in studying the oral aspects of bolus preparation and bolus transfer. These characteristics render ultrasound as highly useful for children or when multiple studies are required to make a diagnosis.

In ultrasound studies of swallowing, a handheld transducer is placed submentally and is rotated 90 degrees. The swallowing functions of the upper surface of the tongue, the intrinsic tongue muscles, and the soft tissue anatomy of the mouth are within the view of the transducer. Ultrasonography does not require the use of any special bolus or contrast; real food can be used. If dysphagia due to pharyngeal or laryngeal dysfunction is suspected, ultrasound offers little diagnostic or treatment information.

Magnetic Resonance Imaging

High speed **magnetic resonance imaging** (MRI), such as **fast low angle shot** (FAST) or **echoplanar imaging,** has allowed a dynamic analysis of the pharyngeal phase of swallowing that was impossible using conventional MRI. The pharyngeal oral cavity, laryngeal lumen, and musculature can be evaluated during motion, allowing the assessment of the swallowing mechanism.

During a fast low angle shot MRI, images are obtained as a bolus containing a contrast substance is swallowed. This technique is particularly useful for assessing rapid activity of the oral cavity.

Magnetic resonance imaging has the advantage of not involving exposure to radiation. However, temporal and spatial resolution of MRI is inferior to videofluroscopy, producing images with poor resolution. Magnetic resonance imaging is costly, and swallowing in the supine position may not reflect the true physiological mechanism of swallowing.

Other Radiographic Tests for Dysphagia

Upper Gastrointestinal Series. Table 5–7 summarizes the testing for dysphagia and gastroesophageal reflux. The single-contrast esophagram study fills and distends the lumen with thin liquid barium. Intrinsic mural irregularities and masses and extrinsic impressions are

Table 5–7. Diagnostic tests of dysphagia and gastroesophageal reflux.*

Test	Indication
• Barium esophagram	• Structural lesions
• Videoradiography	• Pharyngeal function
• Scintigraphy	• Aspiration
• Endoscopic ultrasound	• Submucosal lesions
• Endoscopy	• Structural and mucosal lesions
• Esophageal manometry	• Motility disorders
• 24-hour pH-metry	• Gastroesophageal reflux

*Adapted from Padda and Young[11]

visible. An air-contrast study provides the same information but also allows a more detailed view of the mucosa. For an air-contrast barium study, the patient ingests effervescent crystals followed by thick barium. A barium swallow has both dynamic and static components. The dynamic portion, fluoroscopy, can be recorded on tape (videofluoroscopy, cineradiography) for later review. The static portion is recorded on a series of rapid still frames.

The barium swallow can identify intrinsic and extrinsic pathology (Figure 5–7 to Figure 5–11). Intrinsic abnormalities include tumors, cricopharyngeal dysfunction, aspiration of barium into the airway or reflux into the nasopharynx, diverticula, webs, and esophageal dysmotility. Extrinsic masses such as cervical osteophytes (as seen in Figure 5–10) and an enlarged thyroid gland may be visualized directly or suspected by their effect on the barium column.

The subjective location of dysphagia does not always correspond to the anatomic location of pathology. Therefore, the barium study, when used to evaluate dysphagia, should extend as low as the gastric fundus or cardia. The upper GI series evaluates the stomach and small bowel. Obstruction or dysfunction of these areas may cause or contribute to esophageal dysfunction (e.g., gastroesophageal reflux). Thus, the traditional barium swallow evaluates the upper aerodigestive tract between the oral cavity or oropharynx and the gastric fundus or cardia. It is not intended to identify swallow dysfunction, nor to dictate treatment as in the modified barium swallow.

Computed Tomography and Magnetic Resonance Imaging. **Computed tomography** (CT) and **magnetic resonance imaging** (MRI) are used to delineate the anatomy of a particular region of the head, neck, or other components of the upper aerodigestive tract. The most common use is to identify a site of lesion, such as cerebrovascular accident

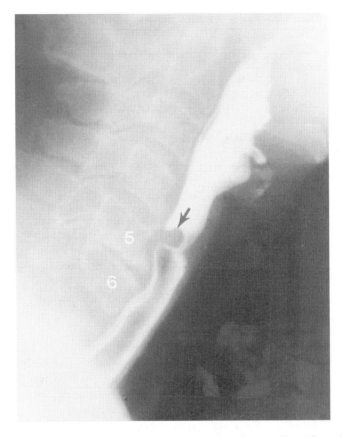

Figure 5–7. Cricopharyngeal dyssynergy. Lateral view of a barium swallow shows the impression of a prominent cricopharyngeus muscle (arrow) on the barium column. An osteophyte at C5–6 (5, 6) causes a smaller impression. Adapted from Weissman JL. Chapter 11. In: Carrau RL, Murry T, eds. *Comprehensive Management of Swallowing Disorders.* San Diego, Calif: Singular Publishing Group; 1999:67.

within the central nervous system, or to delineate the extent of an intra/extraluminal space occupying lesion. In general, CT offers direct axial and coronal images that better define the bony anatomy. Magnetic resonance imaging better delineates the soft tissue (i.e., brain, other neural structures, muscle) in sagittal, coronal, and axial planes but takes longer to complete the images and thus is more prone to motion artifact. Magnetic resonance imaging is more costly than CT.

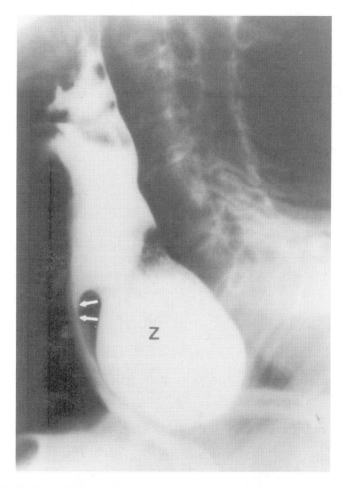

Figure 5–8. Zenker's diverticulum. Oblique view of the cervicothoracic junction shows a large Zenker's diverticulum (Z) that arises above a prominent cricopharyngeus muscle that narrows the barium column (*arrows*). The diverticulum fills completely, and its walls are smooth. From Weissman JL. Chapter 11. In: Carrau RL, Murry T, eds. *Comprehensive Management of Swallowing Disorders.* San Diego, Calif: Singular Publishing Group; 1999:68.

Direct Laryngoscopy

Endoscopy of the upper aerodigestive tract is recommended to rule out or biopsy a neoplasm that may be suspected to be the cause of dysphagia or odynophagia. Occasionally, the endoscopy may be part of the treatment, as in those patients requiring injection of a paralyzed vocal fold, injection of botulinum toxin, or dilation of the esophagus for the treatment of cricopharyngeal achalasia or strictures.

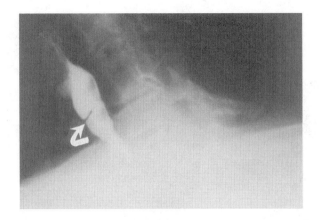

Figure 5–9. Esophageal web. Lateral view of the hypopharynx and cervical esophagus shows the thin, smooth, linear web arising from the anterior wall of the cervical esophagus (*arrow*). There is no obstruction to the flow of barium. From Weissman JL. Chapter 11. In: Carrau RL, Murry T, eds. *Comprehensive Management of Swallowing Disorders.* San Diego, Calif: Singular Publishing Group; 1999:69.

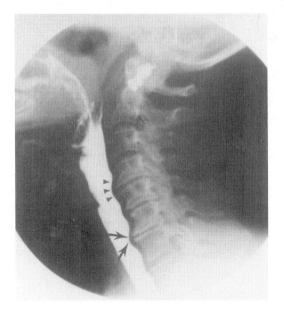

Figure 5–10. Osteophytes ("spurs"). Lateral view of a barium swallow shows anterior cervical osteophytes indenting the posterior wall of the barium-filled cervical esophagus at C6–7 (*arrows*). Anterior disk bulges or nonmineralized osteophytes also deform the barium column (*arrowheads*). From Weissman JL. Chapter 11. In: Carrau RL, Murry T, eds. *Comprehensive Management of Swallowing Disorders.* San Diego, Calif: Singular Publishing Group; 1999:69.

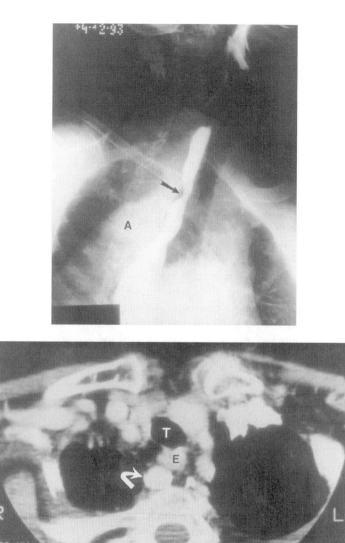

(A)

(B)

Figure 5–11. Aberrant retroesophageal right subclavian artery (dysphagia lusoria). (A) Oblique view of the thoracic esophagus shows a smooth indentation (*arrow*) on the posterolateral wall of the esophagus just above the aortic arch (A). Under fluoroscopic observation, this indentation by the aberrant retroesophageal right subclavian artery pulsated. (B) Axial CT scan shows an aberrant retroesophageal right subclavian artery (*arrow*) passing behind the esophagus (E) and trachea (T). From Weissman JL. Chapter 11. In: Carrau RL, Murry T, eds. *Comprehensive Management of Swallowing Disorders.* San Diego, Calif: Singular Publishing Group; 1999:70.

Esophagoscopy/Gastroscopy

Dysphagia and odynophagia are common indications for upper GI endoscopy and may be performed as the initial test in the evaluation of these disorders. The esophagus is intubated under direct visualization of the posterior hypopharynx. The endoscope is usually advanced through the upper esophageal sphincter, which appears as a slit-like opening in the cricopharyngeus muscle at about 20 cm from the incisor teeth. The entire length of the esophagus is in direct view of the endoscope until its termination at the gastroesophageal junction, which lies at the diaphragmatic hiatus. The esophagus is usually closed at the gastroesophageal junction, but this is easily distended with air insufflation. This allows the endoscope to easily advance through the lower esophageal sphincter into the stomach.

Upper GI flexible endoscopy is the most specific test for identifying esophageal complications of gastroesophageal reflux, esophageal ulcers, infectious disorders, and benign and malignant neoplasms. It is, however, more useful in defining the cause of disease in those patients with solid food dysphagia (transit dysphagia). Absolute contraindications for endoscopy include suspected perforation of the GI tract, lack of adequately trained personnel, and lack of informed consent.

Endoscopic Ultrasound

Endoscopic ultrasound is especially important in the evaluation of submucosal lesions, which cannot be adequately assessed with standard endoscopic techniques (Figure 5–12). Throughout the GI tract, the wall layer echo structure is examined endosonographically.

Intraluminal probes are invasive and thus are not tolerated by all patients. The use of ultrasound intraluminal probes requires a high degree of experience, and sometimes the probe cannot be passed through a tight stricture. **Endoluminal ultrasonography** has been used for the study of esophageal and cricopharyngeal diseases, including esophagitis, strictures, and motility disorders.

Scintigraphy

Scintigraphy is a procedure used to track movement of the bolus and quantify the residual bolus in the oropharynx, pharynx, larynx, and trachea. The patient swallows a small amount of a radionuclide material (such as technetium-99m) combined with liquid or food. A special camera (gamma camera) records images of the organs of interest over time to obtain a quantitative image of the transit and metabolic aspects.

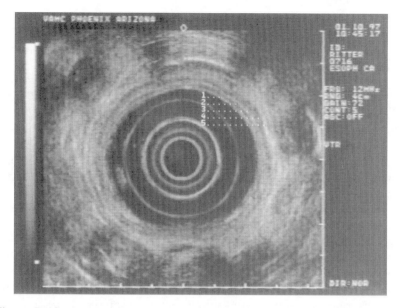

Figure 5–12. A photograph of an endoscopic ultrasound image taken in the esophagus. Layer *1* depicts the superficial mucosa, layer *2* is the deep mucosa, layer *3* corresponds to the submucosa, layer *4* corresponds to the muscularis propria, and layer *5* corresponds to surrounding fat in the esophagus, as there is no serosa in the esophagus. From Padda S, Young MA. Chapter 13. In: Carrau RL, Murry T, eds. *Comprehensive Management of Swallowing Disorders.* San Diego, Calif: Singular Publishing Group; 1999:82.

Scintigraphy can be used to identify trace aspiration and quantify the aspiration over short or long periods of time. Scintigraphy can also be used to calculate the transit time and residual "pooling" of a bolus, before and after treatment, in patients suffering degenerative neuromuscular diseases.

Scintigraphy is typically performed in the nuclear medicine test suite by trained personnel. Acquisition of data from the oral cavity to the thoracic and even upper abdominal cavities may be dynamic during the swallow and then followed by static images over longer time periods, ranging from several minutes to several hours.

The precise amount of aspiration or residual bolus may be identified through computer analysis of the scans made at various time intervals. With the use of scintigraphy, the amount of aspirate in each region may be quantified. Scintigraphy may be more sensitive than barium swallow or modified barium swallow studies for long-term assessment of bolus location, and it has the added advantage of permitting the use of common food as the bolus.

Scintigraphy requires cooperation from the patient. Patients with known movement disorders, severe cognitive disorders, and the inability to remain standing or sitting in front of the gamma camera may not be candidates for this test.

Esophageal pH Monitoring

Prolonged (24-hour) esophageal pH monitoring is the most reliable test for diagnosing GERD. The sensitivity of the test in diagnosing GERD is approximately 90%. In addition, ambulatory monitoring devices permit evaluation of the temporal relationship between reflux episodes and atypical symptoms. pH monitoring is especially important in the diagnostic evaluation of patients with atypical presentations of GERD. Although this is the most reliable test, it is relatively expensive, not available at all institutions, and may not be tolerated by some patients. Dual pH monitoring is now the accepted protocol for identifying esophageal and gastroesophageal reflux. The tests available for assessment of reflux vary. The identification of lesions that may be caused by gastroesophageal reflux requires direct examination (i.e., laryngoscopy, esophagoscopy), while pH monitoring identifies and quantifies the gastroesophageal reflux.

Twenty-four-hour pH monitoring is usually done following an overnight fast. The pH catheter is inserted transnasally into the esophagus. Standard placement of the distal probe is at a position that is approximately 5 cm above the proximal border of the lower esophgeal sphincter. It is ultimately attached to a recording device. Patients are asked to record in a diary, or in the recording device, the times that they eat, sleep, or perform any other activities. More importantly, patients will be asked to record any type of discomfort that they have, including heartburn, chest pain, wheezing, and coughing, and to record the time that these symptoms occurred. This information will be used to correlate the pH at the time a symptom or activity took place, and a symptom index can be calculated.

The most valuable discrimination between physiological and pathologic reflux is the percentage of total time that the pH is less than 4. Normal values for the proximal probe have not yet been established.

Electromyography

Electromyography is the measurement of electrical activity within a muscle. An **electromyogram** (EMG) is recommended to ascertain the presence of specific nerve or neuromuscular unit deficit, such as that

Table 5–8. Electrodiagnostic findings with vocal cord paralysis.*

EMG Findings	Mild		Severity of Injury Moderate		Severe	
Motor unit recruitment	↓↓/↓†	NL	↓↓/NF	↓/↓↓	NF	NF
Motor unit configuration	NL	NL	NL	NL or Poly	0	0
Fibrillations	0	0	+	+	++/+++	CRDs +/++
Prognosis for recovery	Excellent		Favorable		Poor	
Surgical recommendations	No surgery		No permanent surgery. Consider voice therapy and/or Gelfoam injection thyroplasty.		Perform permanent corrective surgery by 6 months.	

*Adapted from Munin and Rainer.[12]
†Key: Recruitment range from Normal (NL), mildly decreased (↓), moderated to decreased with repetitive firing (↓↓) , and nonfiring motor unit (NF). Configuration includes normal (NL), polyphasic potentials with increased duration (Poly), and none (0) to abundant (↓↓↓). CRDs complex repetitive discharges and signify chronic denervation. >21 days describes an EMG evaluation performed on or after 21 days postparalysis. 6 months refers to an EMG study performed no later than 6 months postparalysis. Surgical recommendations assume appropriate workup has been performed.

accompanying vocal fold paralysis or to elucidate or corroborate the presence of a systemic myopathy or degenerative neuromuscular disease. When used for the diagnosis of vocal fold paralysis, a laryngeal EMG may also provide information regarding the prognosis for spontaneous recovery (see Table 5–8).

The goals of a laryngeal EMG are to detect normal from abnormal activity and localize and assess the severity of a focal lesion by determining whether there is **neuro-apraxia** (physiological nerve block or focal injury with intact nerve fibers) or **axonotmesis** (damage to nerve fibers leading to complete peripheral degeneration). A laryngeal EMG can also evaluate prognosis, providing valuable information to either proceed to definitive surgical correction for a permanent or long-term deficit or implement temporary measures if spontaneous recovery is likely.

The thyroarytenoid muscle is approached by insertion of a monopolar or concentric electrode through the cricothryoid ligament

midline 0.5 cm to 1.0 cm, then angled superiorly 45 degrees and laterally 20 degrees for a total depth of 2 cm. The cricothryoid muscle is
reached by inserting the electrode 0.5 cm off the midline, then angling
superiorly and laterally 20 degrees toward the inferior border of the
thyroid cartilage. Figure 5–13 shows a normal recruitment pattern.

Reduced motor unit recruitment is observed with focal demyeli-
nating (neuropraxic) lesions such as found after intubation injuries (Figure 5–14). Patients with axon-loss lesions, such as partial nerve transection after surgical procedures, will also exhibit decreased motor unit
recruitment with normal configuration within the first 6 weeks after
injury. However, axonal injuries will exhibit positive waves and fibrilla-
tion potentials at rest, which begin 3 to 4 weeks postinjury. Laryngeal
nerve regeneration following axon-loss lesions can be observed
between 6 weeks to 12 months postinjury and is characterized by
polyphasic motor unit potentials with wide duration (Figure 5–15).

A laryngeal EMG is useful in differentiating neurologic vocal cord
paralysis from laryngeal joint injury. It may also confirm the diagnosis
of joint dislocation when a normal recruitment pattern is seen with
vocal cord immobility.

The 3 areas of interest for electrodiagnostic evaluation of swallowing are the laryngeal sphincter, the sensory ability of the supraglottic
larynx and pharynx, (indirectly evaluated through cricothyroid muscle
function) and the cricopharyngeal sphincter.

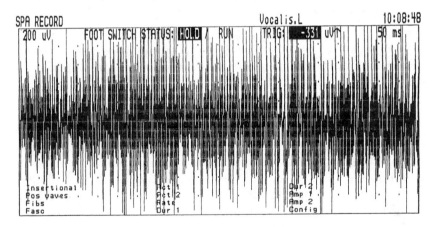

Figure 5–13. Normal voluntary motor unit recruitment of the vocalis muscle using Valsalva's maneuver. Note the full interference pattern that obliterates individual motor unit
analysis when the sweep speed is set at 50 ms per division. From Munin MC, Rainer M.
Chapter 14. In: Carrau RL, Murry T, eds. *Comprehensive Management of Swallowing Disorders.* San Diego, Calif: Singular Publishing Group; 1999:88.

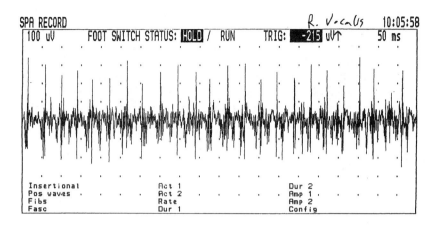

Figure 5–14. Decreased motor unit recruitment with the primary unit firing at 24 Hz. Note that there is a decreased interference pattern with Valsalva's maneuver. The sweep speed is 50 ms/division. From Munin MC, Rainer M. In: Carrau RL, Murry T, eds. *Comprehensive Management of Swallowing Disorders.* San Diego, Calif: Singular Publishing Group; 1999:89.

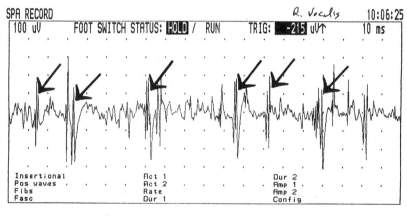

Figure 5–15. Polyphasic motor units are indicated by the arrows. These units do not exhibit typical triphasic configuration and indicate that reinnervation following an axon-loss lesion has occurred. The sweep speed is 10 ms/division. From Munin MC, Rainer M. Chapter 14. In: Carrau RL, Murry T, eds. *Comprehensive Management of Swallowing Disorders.* San Diego, Calif: Singular Publishing Group; 1999:89.

Electromyography, however, has several pitfalls: the precise site of the lesion cannot be determined, except whether it involves the vagus nerve or brainstem, the superior laryngeal nerve, or the recurrent laryngeal nerve. The posterior cricoarytenoid, which is the main abductor muscle, can be technically difficult to localize. Systemic neuromuscular diseases cannot be differentiated from focal lesions without full neurologic evaluation in conjunction with EMG studies of other muscles and nerves.

Pulse Oximetry

A relatively new approach to monitoring swallowing and possibly detecting aspiration is **pulse oximetry.** Pulse oximetry is suggested by some as a well-tolerated and inexpensive option to endoscopy and videofluoroscopy.[13] Pulse oximetry for identifying aspiration is based on the principle that reduced and oxygenated hemoglobin exhibit different absorption characteristics to red and infrared light emitted from a finger or ear probe. Pulse oximetry is noninvasive, simple, and may be repeated often. Pulse oximetry readily measures oxygen desaturation of arterial blood, a condition which is thought to occur as a result of aspiration. Thus, although this test does not provide diagnostic information to formulate treatment plans, it may offer information regarding the presence and possibly the severity of aspiration. This test may be adjunctively used with the bedside swallow evaluation. It is useful in patients who cannot easily be transferred, whose cognition is suspect, or who are in nursing homes where radiological or endoscopic instrumental examinations are not possible. Their technique has yet to be thoroughly tested on multiple populations. Nonetheless, it offers promise to a group of patients who might not otherwise be available for instrumental assessment.

REFERENCES

1. Splaingard M, Hutchins B, Sultan L, Chaudhuri G. Aspiration in rehabilitation patients: videofluoroscopic vs. bedside clinical assessment. *Arch Phys Med Rehabil.* 1988; 69: 637–640.
2. Carrau RL. In: Carrau RL, Murry T, eds. *Comprehensive Management of Swallowing Disorders.* San Diego, Calif: Singular Publishing Group; 1999:33–35.
3. Simonian MA, Goldberg AN. In: Carrau RL, Murry T, eds. *Comprehensive Management of Swallowing Disorders.* San Diego, Calif: Singular Publishing Group; 1999:368.

4. Daniels SK, McAdam CP, Brailey K, Fundas AL. Clinical assessment of swallowing and prediction of dysphagia severity. *Am J Speech Lang Pathol.* 1997; 6:17–23.
5. Logemann JA. *Evaluation and Treatment of Swallowing Disorders.* San Diego, Calif: College Hill Press; 1983.
6. DePippo KL, Hitdas MH, Redding MJ. Validation of the 3 oz water swallow test for aspiration following stroke. *Arch Neurol.* 1992;49:1259–1261.
7. DePippo KL, Holas MA, Redding MJ. The Burke Dysphagia Screening Test: validation of its use in patients with stroke. *Arch Phys Med Rehabil.* 1994;75:1284–1286.
8. Odderson JR, McKenna BA. A model for management of patients with stroke during the acute phase: outcome and economic implications. *Stroke.* 1993;12:1823–1827.
9. Rosenbek JC, Robbins J, Roeker EB, Coyle JL, Woods JL. A penetration-aspiration scale. *Dysphagia.* 1996;11:93–98.
10. Langmore SE, Schatz K, Olsen N. Fibro-optic endoscopic examination of swallowing safety: a new procedure. *Dysphagia.* 1988;2:216–219.
11. Padda S, Young MS. In: Carrau RL, Murry T, eds. *Comprehensive Management of Swallowing Disorders.* San Diego, Calif: Singular Publishing Group; 1999:48.
12. Munin MC, Rainer M. In: Carrau RL, Murry T, eds. *Comprehensive Management of Swallowing Disorders.* San Diego, Calif: Singular Publishing Group; 1999:90.
13. Collins MJ, Bakheit AM. Does pulse oximetry reliably detect aspiration in dysphagic stroke patients? *Stroke.* 1997;28:1773–1775.

Nonsurgical Treatment of Swallowing Disorders

INTRODUCTION

Once the evaluation of the swallowing disorder is completed, a treatment plan is developed and carried out by multiple members of the dysphagia team. As in the diagnostic evaluation, the treatment initially focuses on swallow safety, the prevention of aspiration. The clinicians rely on multiple approaches to swallow safety. These include diet modification; prosthetic management with dental, palatal, or tongue prostheses; direct swallowing therapy; indirect swallowing therapy; and modification of utensils to improve and control feeding. The team members directly involved in the implementation of these techniques include the speech and language pathologist, the maxillofacial prosthodontist, the occupational therapist, the dietitian, the nurse, and the attending physician. Others such as the radiologist, the gastroenterologist, the nurse, and family members may also be involved when there is a need to evaluate additional therapeutic methods or to play a role in the feeding or the observation of feeding. Treatment is a team effort to assure swallow safety, improve nutrition, and contribute to the overall rehabilitative process. As treatment implies change, the clinician must maintain a high degree of vigilance and monitor changes, both positive and negative. To do so requires accurate understanding of the disorder, acute observational skills for the bedside swallow assessment, and the experience and judgment to decide whether or not to use instrumental assessments as part of the decision-making process during treatment.

PROSTHETIC MANAGEMENT
SWALLOWING DISORDERS

Oral prosthodontics is the science of providing suitable substitutes for structures in the oral cavity. Prostheses are used for two main etiologic factors: (1) congenital defects and (2) acquired defects. **Congenital defects** of the oral cavity include cleft lip, cleft palate, cleft mandible, and bifid uvula. **Acquired defects** of the oral cavity are those primarily related to surgical treatment of diseases, traumas, neoplasms, or burns. This section focuses on swallowing disorders related to acquired defects. Prosthetic management of the oral cavity has long been advocated to improve speech intelligibility following limited or extensive surgery to the mandible, maxilla, tongue, or palate. Similarly, prosthetic appliances also serve to improve the oral preparatory and oral phases of swallowing through improvement of chewing, decreasing the tongue-palate distance, and increasing the propulsive pressure on the bolus.

Dentition Enhances Mastication

Adequate dentition may be the difference between a liquid-only diet and a diet that includes both liquids and food consistencies. The **dental prosthesis** may consist of dentures only or may be a combined dental and palatal reshaping as shown in Figure 6–1. The use of teeth or a dental and palatal reshaping prosthesis to grind food to a bolus consistency is a major factor in the types of food one can swallow. A full upper and lower dental arch improves mastication even when oral muscles are weak or partially missing following oral cancer surgery.

Palatal Lowering Prostheses

Hard palate prostheses are devices that help to complement the palatal vault with remaining tongue movement. This helps to increase bolus transit to the posterior oral cavity and increases the tongue-palate contact pressures to propel the bolus into the oropharynx. The palatal lowering prosthesis is designed by the maxillofacial prosthodontist along with the help of the speech and language pathologist to maximize both speech and the oral preparatory and oral phases of swallowing.[1]

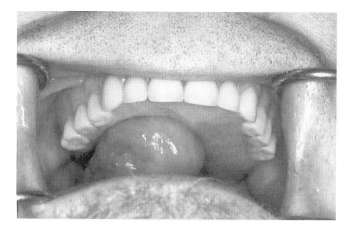

Figure 6–1. Palatal augmentation prostheses with anterior dental prosthesis attached to remaining permanent dentition. From Zaki HS. Dental prosthetics. In: Carrau RL, Murry T, eds. *Comprehensive Management of Swallowing Disorders.* San Diego, Calif: Singular Publishing Group; 1999:253.

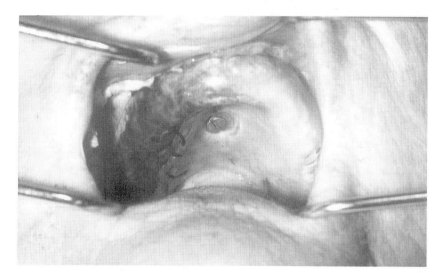

Figure 6–2. Surgical obturator of the hard palate secured with a screw to the remaining hard palate. In Carrau RL, Murry T, eds. *Comprehensive Management of Swallowing Disorders.* San Diego, Calif: Singular Publishing Group; 1999:252.

Prosthetic restoration for swallowing disorders related to surgical defects of the hard palate usually begins with the use of a temporary obturating prosthesis, often inserted in the operating room or shortly thereafter. Figure 6–2 shows a palatal prosthesis fitted with a surgical screw.

After 5 to 7 days, the surgical obturator is removed and remodeled to fit the surgical defect. The obturator restores oronasal separation facilitating oral feedings and speech intelligibility. Restoring the oronasal separation reduces the likelihood of wound infection from residual food particles.

The temporary palatal prosthesis may be substituted for a permanent device several months after surgery. With adequate retention and stability, the prosthesis will provide important intraoral contouring that aids the tongue in the manipulation of the food bolus (oral preparatory and oral phases).

Soft Palate Prostheses

Soft palate prostheses are designed to reduce the distance between the palate and the posterior tongue. If the defect is large, extension of the prosthesis into the pharynx facilitates the sphincteric action of the lateral and posterior pharyngeal wall as shown in Figure 6–3.

Restoration of the soft palate for improved swallowing is recommended when there are large defects involving the posterior border of the soft palate, when there is a nonfunctional band of tissue in the posterior soft palate, or when lateral pharyngeal defects affect the sphincteric action of the palate in conjunction with the tongue and pharynx.

Proper fitting of a hard or soft palate prosthesis should result in improvement of the oral preparatory and oral phases of swallowing. Improvement is based upon shaping the cavity for maximal control of the bolus, maintaining the bolus in the oral cavity without spillage, proper mastication of the bolus, directing the bolus to the posterior oral cavity, slowing down the transit of liquids, and increasing the force of propulsion by reducing the area of defect and bringing the soft palate, or prosthesis, in contact with the remaining tongue. Exercises to complement prosthetic restoration are presented in later paragraphs.

Lingual Prostheses

Partial or total ablative surgery of the tongue (glossectomy) results in significant speech and swallowing disorders. Leonard and Gillis[2] demonstrated improved control of the food bolus using a tongue prosthesis. Total **glossectomy** results in a larger oral cavity where pooling of saliva and liquids can occur. This may ultimately cause postswallow aspiration. Table 6–1 lists the goals of prosthetic rehabilitation after total glossectomy. All these factors play a role in the recovery of swallowing function. The results of a properly fitted tongue prosthesis reduce the oral cavity size, thus reducing the possibility of retained

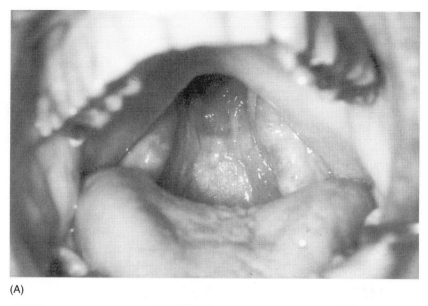

(A)

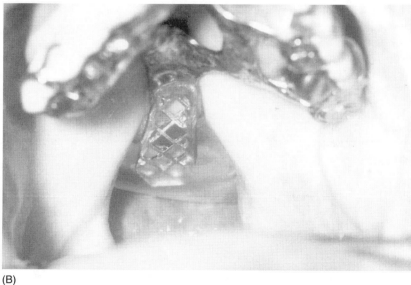

(B)

Figure 6–3. (A) Soft palate prosthesis involving the posterior border of soft palate and (B) with obturator extending into pharyngeal area. Carrau RL, Murry T, eds. *Comprehensive Management of Swallowing Disorders*. San Diego, Calif: Singular Publishing Group; 1999:250.

Table 6–1. Major goals in prosthetic rehabilitation after total glossectomy.*

- To reduce the size of the oral cavity, which will minimize the degree of pooling of saliva and improve speech
- To develop surface contact with the surrounding structures during speech and swallowing
- To protect the underlying fragile mucosa
- To direct the food bolus into the oropharynx
- To improve appearance and psychosocial adjustment

*Adapted from Zaki.[3]

Table 6–2. Treatment to improve swallowing following glossectomy or partial glossectomy.

- Tilt head posteriorly if anterior-posterior tongue movement is impaired. This increases the speed of oral transit.
- Tilt head to the side least affected to control movement of bolus.
- Thermal stimulation may assist in activating the pharyngeal swallow by increasing sensation near the anterior faucial pillars.
- Tongue palate contact exercises with specific placement goals may strengthen the posterior tongue movement or increase the range of posterior tongue motion.
- Use chewing exercises manipulating wet gauze or chewing gum to practice manipulating the bolus.
- Practice speech sounds such as *d, t, g,* and *k* to improve range of motion of remaining structures.

secretions that might later be aspirated. The speech and language pathologist must help the patient to direct foods and liquids into the pharynx to gain the maximum benefit. This may require use of a syringe to place food posteriorly or having the patient monitor placement by eating in front of a mirror.

The treatment of swallowing following cancer that requires glossectomy includes the procedures outlined in Table 6–2. The patient with total glossectomy will require management from many members of the dysphagia team, including those who can develop feeding devices to aid in the oral preparatory and oral phases of swallowing.

INDIRECT SWALLOWING THERAPY

Indirect swallowing therapy consists of exercises to strengthen control of the voluntary oral preparatory and oral phases of swallowing. In addition, this therapy includes methods to stimulate the pharyngeal swallow and to increase protective valving at the level of the vocal folds to prevent aspiration. Thus, indirect swallowing therapy involves exercises for the organs of swallowing without requiring the patient to swallow foods or liquids. Numerous studies have provided limited evidence that indirect techniques are useful in the management of dysphagia. However, it should be pointed out that most of the evidence to support the use of indirect swallowing therapy was obtained from small groups of patients. Moreover, in many of the groups studied, spontaneous improvement or recovery of the oral swallowing function was expected, such as in patients with limited CVA. Indirect swallowing therapy is indicated in patients who demonstrate

1. Adequate cognitive skills to follow instruction
2. Motivation to improve
3. Willingness to practice independently
4. A need to increase muscle strength, range of motion, or sensory awareness as indicated by modified barium swallow or fiberoptic endoscopic evaluation of swallowing testing

Oral Motor Exercises

Oral motor exercises have long been suggested as a way to increase control of the oral phase of swallowing by increasing volitional control over the movements of lips, tongue, and vocal folds. Many of these exercises are derived from the speech and voice rehabilitation literature based on the treatment of dysarthria. Since dysarthric speech and voice generally improve when the patient controls the movements of the articulators, the rationale for use of oral motor exercises to treat swallowing disorders is to slow the passage of the bolus, increase awareness of the bolus, and maximize the driving force of the bolus in transit to the oropharynx.

Control of the lips is addressed in order to maintain the bolus in the oral cavity. Labial exercises improve strength of closure, symmetry of closure, and awareness of closure. Table 6–3 lists common labial exercises. These may be done during the indirect treatment of swallowing or used in conjunction with direct swallowing therapy.

Table 6–4 summarizes exercises for the tongue and mandible. For patients with trismus, exercises to increase mouth opening using a device such as the Therabite® allows the clinician and the patient to set

Table 6–3. Labial exercises to improve strength and awareness of control of the swallowing mechanism.*

1. Rapid labial opening and closing using the consonants /p, b/.
2. Extended lip squeeze followed by lip retraction.
3. Repeating the vowels /u, i/ with increased lip movement. Vocalization provides additional stimulation and awareness.
4. Thermal stimulation of the lips with ice. Movement of the ice may be medial-lateral or more focal if drooling on one side is prevalent.
5. Holding different objects between the lips such as a straw, tongue blade, plastic spoon, and so on, to improve sensory awareness. Objects may be of different sizes, shapes, and weights.
6. Apply various foods to lips such as yogurt and peanut butter, and encourage the patient to massage the lips together.
7. Use the index finger to apply a sudden or quick stretch to the edges of the upper and lower lips.
8. Practice humming. Cue patient to start and stop humming. When humming stops, the patient should open the lips, then close again.
9. Have patient close the lips. Ask him or her to keep them closed while you try gently to break the lip seal.
10. Practice a "facial squeeze" by squeezing lips together. While keeping lips closed, alternate bringing teeth together and separating them. This mimics chewing activity.
11. Practice inhaling and exhaling through the nose rather than the mouth. The patient may want to watch this activity with a mirror.
12. Prior to swallowing, the patient should hold a glass or cup to the lips. Practice the timing of opening the lips once the cup is placed on the lower lip.
13. Hold a small object such as a button (connected to a string) and place it between the lips and teeth. The clinician can put a gentle pull on the string to improve lip strength.
14. Intraoral stimulation of cheeks with a brush, cold object, or fingers.
15. Resistive exercises. Example: have the patient push the upper lip down while the clinician resists the movement with a tongue blade. Have the patient push the tongue against the cheek while the clinician resists against the outside of the cheek.

*Adapted from Murry.[4]

goals and monitor progress. For those patients who successfully increase their mouth opening, the improved placement of food may significantly enhance swallowing, especially if surgery has caused alterations of the anatomy. It also expands the choices of foods, often obviating the need for special diets just for the sole purpose of accommodating a restricted oral opening.

Vocal fold closure is a key factor in preventing aspiration. When the vocal folds fail to close for a sufficient amount of time, the risk of aspiration increases. Along with techniques listed here, the exercises in Table 6–5 provide indirect strategies for stimulating increased vocal

Table 6–4. Exercises for tongue and mandible strength and movement.*

1. Tongue tip elevation. Place tongue tip on alveolar ridge. Hold it for 2 seconds.
2. Tongue tip sweep. After holding the tongue on the alveolar ridge, sweep posteriorly against the palate.
3. Use the phonemes /t, d/ for rapid contact and release of the tongue tip to the alveolar ridge.
4. Use the "ch" sound to improve tongue contact to the middle of the soft palate. Similarly, the sounds s and sh help with lateral contact of tongue to palate as well as help to groove the tongue.
5. The /k, g/ phonemes are used to increase posterior tongue to soft palate contact. Combining syllables into quick movements such as "ta-ka" or "cha-ka" is helpful to improve the sweeping motion of the tongue.
6. Range of motion exercises can be done by chewing on gauze, initially, then adding small amounts of food when it is safe.
7. To improve sensory awareness, use pressure and temperature stimulation.
   a. A cold spoon may be placed on the tip, blade, or back of tongue. Light pressure is applied, and the patient is asked to lift the spoon.
   b. The palate is touched with tongue blade or cotton, and the patient is asked to touch the area with the tongue.
   c. Cold or sour materials are given to the patient. They may be frozen on a stick if the patient is not yet cleared to swallow.
   d. Various sizes and textures of bolus may be given to identify the size and texture most easily transported by the tongue.
8. Mandible movement. Patients with reduced mandible movement may want to use a device such as Therabite® to increase mouth opening.
9. Resistive exercises to the mandible such as lowering or closing the mandible against the pressure applied by the therapist on the chin.
10. Sucking exercises increase tongue palate contact and help the patient to manage saliva. Sucking may be done with the tongue tip against the alveolar ridge and lips and teeth slightly apart or with teeth closed using a "slurping" or "suctioning" pull of the tongue to the mid-palate area. The patient should try to do this with as much sound as possible to increase sensory feedback.

*Adapted from Murry.[4]

fold closure. Of specific note is Item 6 in Table 6–5. The **Lee Silverman Voice Treatment** (LSVT) was developed for treating speech intelligibility in Parkinson's patients. Studies by Ramig and her colleagues[5] have validated the efficacy of these exercises. The focus of this treatment is on increasing the valving ability of the vocal folds. Sharkawi et al[6] demonstrated that oral and pharyngeal transit times were reduced significantly. Moreover, after 16 sessions of LSVT, they found a 51% reduction in the numbers of swallowing disorders over various types of boluses.

Table 6–5. Vocal fold closure and laryngeal elevation techniques.*

1. Practice coughing.
2. Increase the loudness of the voice.
3. Initiate voice with a hard glottal onset.
4. Produce sustained phonation. Try to increase the duration while maintaining consistent voice quality.
5. Sustain phonation at various pitches. This helps with anterior vocal fold closure as well as laryngeal elevation.
6. An excellent program of laryngeal exercises has been developed by Ramig and her colleagues.[†] This program is called *Lee Silverman Voice Treatment.* While this program is primarily to increase vocal effectiveness, it also offers promise to those who require increased vocal fold closure to reduce the risk of aspiration.

*Adapted from Murry.[4]
[†]Ramig et al.[5]

Specific impairments may benefit from repetition of specific tasks. Table 6–6 lists 14 common impairments or defects found after the loss of tissue or after neurologic damage, along with the goals and tasks to reach each goal. When the patient focuses on only one or two goals at a time, improvement may be more easily documented and the patient may better understand the goals, thus improving patient motivation to participate in the therapy.

Thermal Stimulation

Thermal stimulation may be defined as the stroking or rubbing of one or more of the organs of swallowing with a cold probe. Rosenbek and others[8] theorized that touch and cold stimulation provide heightened **oral awareness** and an alerting stimulus to the brainstem and brain to trigger the pharyngeal swallow faster than it would without the stimulation. While these authors found slight improvements in the duration of stage transition and the total swallow duration, the amount of time needed to do the stimulation was extensive. To date, there is little research to support the extensive use of cold stimulation to the anterior faucial arches.

Head-Raising Exercise

The **head-raising exercise** is an isotonic/isometric exercise aimed at strengthening muscles that contribute to the opening of the upper esophageal sphincter, specifically, the geniohyoid, thyrohyoid, and digastric muscles.[9] The exercise consists of lying in the supine position and sustaining a head raise for one minute followed by a rest period. If the patient cannot sustain the head for one minute, an alternate baseline time period can be used at the start. The result of this exercise is to increase the swallow-induced anterior excursion of the larynx and to significantly decrease the hypopharyngeal intrabolus pressure, suggesting a decline in pharyngeal outflow resistance.

Oral Motor Exercises: Pros and Cons

Oral motor exercises have been used for years to treat speech disorders. Only recently have these exercises been applied and modified for use in patients with swallowing disorders. Only limited data is available to demonstrate the effectiveness of these exercises. The Agency for Health Care Policy and Research reported on only 4 studies of noninvasive or indirect swallowing therapy. The studies summarized in Table 6–7 suggest that there is only limited evidence that indirect therapy has significant positive effects on clinical outcomes (e.g., reduced pneumonia, weight gain) for patients with neurologic disorders.

For patients who have undergone treatment for head and neck cancer, it appears that indirect noninvasive exercise may also have value. Recent studies by Logeman and colleagues,[14,15,16,17] as well as others such as Dworkin, and Nudal[18] Martin, et al.[19] and Sonies,[20] have shown that active participation in a swallowing rehabilitation program using indirect maneuvers improves swallow function following head and neck surgery.

The use of indirect exercises should be based on anatomic and physiological findings of instrumental and clinical bedside assessments. These exercises may be coupled with prosthetic management and with direct therapies.

It remains to be seen how efficacious the indirect treatment is as a unitary method. The dilemma may never be completely resolved since it would require controlled studies that involve the withholding of treatment for some patients, which may be detrimental to their welfare and therefore unethical. Clinicians must guard against blindly treating patients with indirect swallowing exercises unless they can specify a rationale for treatment and document their effects on swallowing safety, weight gain, and quality of life. Indirect swallowing therapy should be combined with other treatment modalities when the clinician deems it appropriate.

Table 6–6. Exercises related to specific improvements in swallowing.*

Impairment	Goal
Limited control, agility or neck rotation, extension and flexion.	Range, control, agility adequate for needed task.
Trismus. Inability of the jaw to open due to injury to the trigeminal nerve or muscular deficiency.	Adequate opening for feeding route (spoon, fork, cup, or biting), for denture or palatal prosthesis placement, and for oral hygiene.
Weakness or absence of mandibular support/control.	Symmetric mandible-maxilla approximation supportive of potentials for posture, oral nutrition/hydration, and speech.
Weakness or absence of buccal tone.	Increased buccal tone.
Diminished labial opening.	Adequate labial opening size for eating. Adequate shaping for speech.
Partial or complete labial incompetence.	Oral continence for saliva management, eating/drinking, and speech.
Unilateral partial or complete lingual weakness or missing lateral lingual tissue.	Posterior bolus retention-release control for airway protection. Bolus and airflow control (minimize lateral "leaks").
Bilateral lingual weakness.	Oral transit with minimum oral loss. Maximum coordination with initiation of swallow gestures.
Absent tongue.	Development of compensatory mandibular, labial, and head/neck movement strategies.
Unilateral or complete weakness or missing tissue of the palate.	Adequate velopharyngeal closure if tissue is adequate. Effective obturation if tissue is inadequate.
Unilateral, bilateral, or regional failure of pharyngeal constriction.	Improved bolus compression.
Incomplete glottic closure.	Improved glottic closure.
Incomplete supraglottic closure.	Improved supraglottic closure.
Inadequate PRS opening for swallow.	Maximum PES opening.

Table 6–6. *continued*

Tasks May Include

Obtain consult from physical therapy; depending on need, tasks may focus on development of agility of movement as well as control and ROM.

Maintain mandible-maxilla alignment while increasing passive and active range of mandible opening. Movements should be made slowly. Maximum stretch should be maintained ≥ 15 seconds. The Therabite™ is a more sophisticated device, especially useful for marked trismus or when alignment of mandible and maxilla is difficult to maintain.

Establish optimal alignment passively or actively and present exercises graded for endurance. Increase strength and control using graded resistance and biting, munching tasks to strengthen muscles of mandibular closure and opening.

Isometric tightening of the buccal area or squeezing of soft objects between cheek and teeth/gums or from buccal sulcus to the molar surface.

Passive stretching and exercises to increase range and strength of lateral commisure movement. Maintain mandible alignment throughout.

Develop agility for desired range using tasks graded for speed and accuracy. Maintain mandible alignment throughout.

Maximize lingual symmetry at rest and in a variety of nonspeech and speech gestures. Squeezing and lingual manipulation tasks may be appropriate. Palatal prosthesis may facilitate therapy.

Address sectionally, as above.

Develop ROM and agility of movements needed for compensations that take advantage of gravity. Consider mandibular or maxillary shaping prosthesis.

Sustained blowing against resistance may strengthen closure. Endoscopic feedback may be helpful even with obturation. Obturation may actually recruit improved compensatory participation in closure from the lateral and posterior pharyngeal walls.

Maximum lingual retraction. Laryngeal elevation and supraglottic closure.

Attempt to establish conditions, resulting in improved true vocal fold approximation using pitch, positional, compression, and respiratory support strategies while avoiding false vocal fold participation.

Habituate early and effortful laryngeal closure and elevation for swallow. The Mendelsohn manoeuver may be used.

Maximizing extent and timing of hyoid/laryngeal elevation and the effects of pharyngeal compression of the bolus.

*Adapted from Leonard and Kendall.[7]

Table 6–7. Characteristics of controlled studies of noninvasive therapies for dysphagia.

Study	N	Study Design	Care Setting	Mean Age
Groher 1987*	23	RCT	Home nursing	71.8
				74.2
Kasprisin et al 1989†	48	Retro	Hospital	NR
	13	CT		
	8			
Martens et al 1990‡	16	HPCS	Acute hospital unit	49.3
	15			46.1
De Pippo et al 1994§	38	RCT	Rehab unit	76
	38			74.5
	38			73

*Groher.[10]
†Kasprisin et al.[11]
‡Martens et al.[12]
§De Pippo et al.[13]
RCT = randomized controlled trial
CT = controlled trial
HPCS = historical prospective case series
NR = not reported

DIRECT SWALLOWING THERAPY

Direct swallowing therapy involves the use of foods and liquids to practice swallowing techniques, maneuvers, and indirect exercises. Direct therapy is reserved for those who demonstrate, through instrumental studies or other means (such as pulse oximetry, temperature monitoring, etc.) that they can successfully swallow small amounts of food or liquid. While no diagnostic technique—instrumental or otherwise—is perfect at predicting the risk of aspiration, the experienced clinician will be able to combine anatomic, physiological, psychological, and cognitive information with available instrumental and bedside evaluations to prescribe direct therapy and to ascertain the amounts and consistencies of the bolus to be swallowed.

Swallow Maneuvers

The most important maneuvers to upgrade the patient's voluntary control over the various aspects of the pharyngeal swallow and to preserve control of the bolus during the pharyngeal swallow are

Table 6–7. *continued*

Primary Disease(s)	Treatment	Time Frame
CVA with history of aspirtion pneumonia	Pureed diet, mechanically altered diet	6 months
Various	Swallow therapy	NR
Brain injury, tumor, CVA	Various (diet, exercise counseling) No specific dysphagia treatment	NR
CVA	Diet and swallow techique recommendations, therapist-prescribed diet and swallow techniques. Therapist-prescribed diet and techniques reinforced	1 year

1. Supraglottic swallow
2. Super-supraglottic swallow
3. Effortful swallow
4. Mendelsohn maneuver

The **supraglottic swallow** is a 4-step maneuver: (1) inhale and hold breath, (2) place bolus in swallow position, (3) swallow while holding breath, (4) cough after swallow before inhaling. The effect of this maneuver is to close the vocal folds (breath hold) and clear any residue that may have entered the laryngeal vestibule (cough) before breathing again.

The **super-supraglottic swallow** is similar to the supraglottic swallow, with the addition of the instruction to bear down once the breath is being held. The effect of bearing down is to increase false vocal fold closure and assist in closing the posterior glottis.

The **effortful swallow** is simply a squeeze. The patient is instructed to squeeze hard with all of his or her muscles. This maneuver may be the easiest for patients who have trouble following multiple-stage commands, for children, or for those patients with significant sensory loss.

The **Mendelsohn maneuver** is a technique to open the upper esophageal sphincter. In this maneuver, the patient initiates several dry swallows while trying to feel the elevation of the thyroid prominence. Then, the instruction is to hold the larynx up for several seconds. By keeping the larynx tilted and elevated, the upper esophageal sphincter

Table 6–8. Swallow maneuvers.*

Swallow Maneuvers	Problem for Which Maneuver Designed	Rationale
Supraglottic swallow	Reduced or late vocal fold closure	Voluntary breath hold usually closes vocal folds before and during swallow.
	Delayed pharyngeal swallow	Closes vocal folds before and during delay.
Super-supraglottic swallow	Reduced closure of airway entrance	Effortful breath hold tilts arytenoid forward, closing airway entrance before and during swallow.
Effortful swallow	Reduced posterior movement of the tongue base	Effort increases posterior tongue-base movement.
Mendelsohn maneuver	Reduced laryngeal movement	Laryngeal movement opens the upper esophageal sphincter; prolonging laryngeal elevation prolongs upper esophageal sphincter opening.
	Discoordinated swallow	Normalizes timing of pharyngeal swallow events.

From Logemann.[21]

relaxes to allow food to pass, leaving less residual material in the hypopharyngeal area.

Table 6–8 summarizes the swallowing maneuvers, the problems for which they were designed, and the rationale for their use. These maneuvers should be slowly explained to the patient, tried first without foods or liquids (i.e., dry swallow), and then ideally be tested during instrumental studies of swallowing function before recommending them for continuous therapy. They may be tried during the bedside swallow evaluation on a limited basis as a method for determining the patient's ability to perform the tasks during the instrumental examination.

Recently, Lazarus and colleagues[22] demonstrated that the base-of-the-tongue pressures and duration of contact to the posterior pharyngeal wall increased using each of four maneuvers in patients who underwent surgery or radiation for head and neck cancer. This increase was greatest for effortful swallow and tongue-hold swallow. Although they only studied three patients, these preliminary findings suggest that the swallow maneuvers increase the remaining base-of-tongue pressure and the duration of contact.

Swallow Postures

Numerous individuals have demonstrated that by turning the head to one side, by tucking the chin down toward the chest, or by tilting the head back, swallowing can be facilitated or aspiration can be reduced or prevented. Postural adjustments used in direct swallow exercises can reduce aspiration, improve transit times (oral and pharyngeal), and decrease the amount of residue after the swallow.

Table 6–9, adapted from Logemann,[21] reports the specific effects of body postures during fluoroscopy and the rationale for using the specific postures. The importance of teaching the postures prior to the instrumental swallow evaluation is underscored here. Data demonstrating the efficacy of these body postures has been primarily derived from small groups of patients with various neurologic, neuromuscular, and head and neck cancer diagnoses. Each individual patient's ability to improve speech of swallow, reduce pooling, and control aspiration will dictate further treatment. Thus, while all of these techniques have shown efficacy in clinical research studies, the clinician must still continue to rely on his or her clinical judgment as to when to use which technique when treating a patient with a swallowing disorder.

SWALLOWING THERAPY AND ASPIRATION

It is to be expected that patients recovering from swallowing disorders will experience occasional aspiration. The indirect and direct techniques reviewed in this chapter can be efficacious in reducing aspiration events and preventing aspiration pneumonia. A summary of the nonsurgical methods to reduce or eliminate aspiration is shown in Table 6–10. Chapter 7 reviews the surgical controls for reducing or eliminating aspiration.

Table 6–9. Postural techniques to reduce or eliminate aspiration or residue.*

Disorder Observed on Fluoroscopy	Posture Applied
Inefficient oral transit (reduced posterior propulsion of bolus by tongue)	Head back
Delay in triggering the pharyngeal swallow (bolus past ramus of mandible but pharyngeal swallow is not triggered)	Chin down
Reduced posterior motion of tongue-base (residue in valleculae)	Chin down
Unilateral vocal fold paralysis or surgical removal (aspiration during the swallow)	Head rotated to damaged side
Reduced closure of laryngeal entrance and vocal folds (aspiration during the swallow)	Chin down; head rotated to damaged side
Reduced pharyngeal contraction (residue spread throughout pharynx)	Lying down on one side
Unilateral pharyngeal paresis (residue on one side of pharynx)	Head rotated to damaged side
Unilateral oral and pharyngeal weakness on same side (residue in mouth and pharynx on same side)	Head tilt to stronger side
Cricopharyngeal dysfunction (residue in piriform sinuses)	Head rotated

*From Logemann.[21]

Groher[23] suggested that those variables that separate those patients who develop aspiration pneumonia from those who do not remain speculative. Presumably, the number of patients who aspirate is much greater than that of those who develop aspiration pneumonia. Factors such as prior history of aspiration, mobility, age, state of consciousness, respiratory status, upper airway reflexes, results of instrumental swallowing evaluation, and the integrity of the lower airway protective mechanisms all contribute to prevention of aspiration pneu-

Table 6–9. *continued*

Rationale
Uses gravity to clear oral cavity
Widens valleculae to prevent bolus entering airway; narrows airway entrance, reducing risk of aspiration
Pushes tongue-base backward toward pharyngeal wall
Places extrinsic pressure on thyroid cartilage, improving vocal fold approximation, and directs bolus down stronger side
Puts epiglottis in more protective position; narrows laryngeal entrance; improves vocal fold closure by applying extrinsic pressure
Eliminates gravitational effect on pharyngeal residue
Eliminates damaged side of pharynx from bolus path
Directs bolus down stronger side by gravity
Pulls cricoid cartilage away from posterior pharyngeal wall, reducing resting pressure in cricopharyngeal sphincter

monia. Prospective studies of either those postsurgical cases of head and neck cancer, post-CVA or progressive neurologic diseases are ethically questionable. Table 6–11A and Table 6–11B list factors that are associated with or contribute to the risk of aspiration pneumonia. These risk factors must always be tempered with the disease and patient factors for each individual. Clinical judgment suggests that, given a decreased medical condition and enough regular signs of aspiration, one may ultimately expect aspiration pneumonia.

Table 6–10. Nonsurgical methods for controlling aspiration.

Oral Motor Exercises

• Lip seal
• Tongue retraction and elevation
• Tongue strengthening

Head Position Maneuvers

• Chin tuck
• Head lift
• Rotating head to side of lesion in pharyngeal or vocal fold paresis

Postural Compensation Techniques

• Sitting upright
• Lying on side

Swallowing Retraining

• Supraglottic swallow
• Super-supraglottic swallow
• Mendelsohn maneuver
• Multiple swallows
• Frequent throat clearing

Diet Modification

• Change in bolus size
• Change in food consistencies
• Changes in temperature and taste

Non-oral Diet (NPO)

Table 6–11A. Factors contributing to aspiration pneumonia.

• Aspirate
  Nature
  Frequency
  Amount
  Depth
• Oral hygiene/dentition
• Pulmonary reserve
• Nutritional status
• Immune status
• Caretaker

Table 6–11B. Risk factors associated with aspiration pneumonia.

- Dysphagia/aspiration
- Hospitalization
- Oral hygiene
- Dehydration
- Immune compromise
- Cough/ "pulmonary function"
- Presence of a feeding tube
- Bed-bound
- Alertness/cognitive
- Dependent for feeding
- Needs suctioning
- Recent weight loss

REFERENCES

1. Wheeler R, Logemann JA, Rosen M. Maxillary reshaping prostheses: effectiveness in improving speech and swallowing of postsurgical oral cancer patients. *J Prosthet Dent*. 1980;43:313–319.
2. Leonard R, Gillis R. Effects of a prosthetic tongue on vowel intelligibility and food management in a patient with total glossectomy. *J Speech Hear Disord*. 1982,47:25–32.
3. Zaki HS. In: Carrau RL, Murry T, eds. *Comprehensive Management of Swallowing Disorders*. San Diego, Calif: Singular Publishing Group; 1999:252.
4. Murry T. In: Carrau RL, Murry T, eds. *Comprehensive Management of Swallowing Disorders*. San Diego, Calif: Singular Publishing Group; 1999:244–246.
5. Ramig L, Shapiro S, Countryman S, Paulas A, Obrien C, Hoefin M, Thompson L. Intensive voice treatment (LSVT) for individuals with Parkinson's disease: a two-year follow-up. *NCVS Status Prog Rep*. 1999; 14: 131–140.
6. Sharkawi AE, Ramig L, Logemann JA, Pauloski BR, Pawlas A, Baum S, Werner C. Effects of Lee Silverman Voice Treatment on swallow function in patients with Parkinson's disease. Poster: Dysphagia Research Society; October 15–17, 1998; New Orleans, La.
7. Leonard R, Kendall K. *Dysphagia Assessment and Treatment Planning: A Team Approach*. San Diego, Calif: Singular Publishing Group; 1999:187–191.
8. Rosenbek JA, Robbins J, Willford WO, Kirk G, Schlitz A, Sowell TW, Deutsch SE, Milanti FJ, Ashford J, Graminigna GD, Fogarty A, Dong K, Rau MT, Prescott TE, Lloyd AM, Sterkel MT, Hansen JE. Comparing treatment intensities of tactile-thermal application. *Dysphagia*. 1998;13:1–9.

9. Kahrilas PJ, Logemann JA, Krugler C, Flanagan, E. Volitional augmentation of upper esophageal sphincter opening during swallowing. *Am J Physiol.* 1991;260:G450–G456.

10. Groher ME. Bolus management and aspiration pneumonia in patients with pseudo bulbar dysphagia. *Dysphagia.* 1987;1:215–216.

11. Kasprisin AT, Clumeck H, Nino-Morcia M. The efficacy of rehabilitative management of dysphagia. *Dysphagia.* 1989;4:48–52.

12. Martens L, Cameron T, Simonsen M. Effects of a multidisciplinary management program on neurologically impaired patients with dysphagia. *Dysphagia.* 1990;5:147–151.

13. De Pippo KL, Holas MA, Reding MJ, Mandel FS, Lesser ML. Dysphagia therapy following stroke: a controlled trial. *Neurology.* 1994;44:1655–1660.

14. Lazarus CL, Logemann JA, Rademaker AW, Kahrilas PJ, Pajak T, Lazar R, Halper A. Effects of bolus volume, viscosity, and repeated swallows in nonstroke subjects and stroke patients. *Arch Phys Med Rehabil* 1993;74:1066–1070.

15. Lazzara G, Lazarus CL, Logemann JA. Impact of thermal stimulation on the triggering of the swallowing reflex. *Dysphagia.* 1986:73–77.

16. Logemann JA. Evaluation and treatment planning for the head-injured patient with oral intake disorders. *J Head Trauma Rehabil.* 1989;4:113.

17. Logemann JA, Karhilas P, Hurst P, Davis J, Krugler C. Effects of intraoral prosthetics on swallowing in oral cancer patients. *Dysphagia.* 1989;4:118.

18. Dworkin JP, Nadal JC. Nonsurgical treatment of drooling in a patient with closed head injury and severe dysarthria. *Dysphagia.* 1991;6:40–49.

19. Martin BJ, Corlew M, Wood H, Olson D, Golopol L, Wingo M, Kirmani N. The association of swallowing dysfunction and aspiration pneumonia. *Dysphagia.* 1994;9:1–6.

20. Sonies BC. Remediation challenges in treating dysphagia post head/neck cancer: a problem-oriented approach. *Clin Commun Disord.* 1993;3:21–26.

21. Logemann JA. Therapy for oropharyngeal swallowing disorders. In: Perlman AL, Schulze-Delrieu K, eds. Deglutition and Its Disorders. San Diego, Calif: Singular Publishing Group; 1997:451, 455.

22. Lazarus CL, Song C, Logemann JA, Rademaker AW, Kahrilas PJ. Effects of maneuvers on tongue base function for swallowing: a pilot study. Poster: Dysphagia Research Society; October 15–17, 1998; New Orleans, La.

23. Groher M. Risks and benefits of oral feeding. *Dysphagia.* 1994;9:233–235.

CHAPTER

7

Surgical Treatment of Swallowing Disorders

VOCAL FOLD MEDIALIZATION

Medialization of the vocal fold may be effected by using transendoscopic, transoral, or transcutaneous injection or by using open transcervical techniques (Table 7–1).

Vocal Fold Injection

Vocal fold injection lateral to the vocal fold is useful to medialize the vocal fold when it shows atrophy, paresis, or immobility with a prognosis of improvement. Vocal fold medialization from a lateral vocal fold injection improves the closure of the glottis, thus improving swallowing efficiency and safety. Vocal fold injection has the advantage of avoiding open surgery, but it is technically demanding and may present complications, as shown in Table 7–2. Contraindications for vocal fold injection include a compromised airway and/or lack of clear evidence that the dysphagia is secondary to a paralyzed vocal fold.

Gelfoam®, a mixture of gelatin powder with a buffered saline solution, may be used as a temporary treatment of vocal fold paralysis. Gelfoam® injection of the vocal fold can result in improved swallowing and is an excellent option for the treatment of dysphagia due to vocal

Table 7–1. Vocal fold medialization.

Injection

Gelfoam®
Teflon®
Autologous tissue
  Fat
  Fascia
  Collagen

Laryngeal Framework Surgery

Medialization laryngoplasty
  Silastic
  Gortex®
  Hydroxyapatite
  Cartilage
Arytenoid adduction/repositioning

Table 7–2. Complications of vocal fold injection.

- Over-injection: improper vocal fold closure (early anterior contact); airway obstruction.
- Misplaced injection: inappropriate segmental glottic closure.
- Under-injection: lack of vocal fold closure.

---

fold paralysis when the recovery of the vocal fold paralysis is likely. Gelfoam® is reabsorbed within 12 weeks.

    Autologous fat injection has been used as material for the treatment of both voice and swallowing disorders. Its reabsorption is variable, thus making the final result somewhat unpredictable. In a typical injection, the vocal fold is over-injected, thus creating a convex vocal fold, to account for the initial reabsorption of fat. However, this convexity causes early anterior contact and a posterior gap, which may increase the risk of aspiration.

    Teflon® injection is frequently effective in improving vocal function, particularly if the vocal fold is not too far from the midline. However, when the paralyzed vocal fold is in the cadaveric position, Teflon® is not very effective in treating aspiration, and, in addition, voice quality is usually poor. In such patients, a large posterior gap persists after Teflon® injection, even when there appears to be adequate closure of the anterior glottis. Additionally, Teflon® has lost favor as an injectable material for the larynx due to the occurrence of teflon granuloma. The complications and advantages of Teflon® are shown in Table 7–3.

Table 7–3. Intracordal teflon® injection.*

Problems and Complications

- Difficult surgical exposure (e.g., cervical spine limited range of motion)
- Nonreversible
- Technically challenging
- Inconsistent postoperative vocal quality
- Does not close posterior glottic gap
- Teflon® migration
- Teflon® granuloma

Advantages

- Does not require open surgery
- May be performed in an office setting (selected cases)

*Reprinted with permission. Adapted from Andrews et al.[1]

Table 7–4. Silastic medialization laryngoplasty.*

Indications

- Glottic incompetence secondary to unilateral vocal fold paralysis
- Sacrifice of or injury to cranial nerve X during skull base surgery
- Incomplete glottic closure secondary to vocal fold paresis or atrophy
- Selected traumatic or postsurgical defects

Contraindications

Relative
- Fibrosis resulting from laryngeal radiation
- Loss of external framework (i.e., vertical hemilaryngectomy)
- Prior Teflon® injection

Absolute
- Impaired contralateral vocal fold abduction (i.e. airway compromise)

*Reprinted with permission. Adapted from Andrews et al.[1]

LARYNGEAL FRAMEWORK SURGERY

Medialization Laryngoplasty

Medialization laryngoplasty for vocal fold paralysis requires the insertion of an implant between the ala of the thyroid cartilage and the vocal fold. The bulk of the implant medializes the fold and in selected cases may even adduct the vocal process. Table 7–4 lists the most common indications and contraindications for silastic medialization of the

Table 7–5. Advantages and disadvantages of medialization laryngoplasty.*

Advantages

• Well tolerated under local anesthesia
• Reversible and adjustable
• Reproducible vocal results (does not interfere with mucosal wave)
• Can be performed in conjunction with arytenoid adduction (closes posterior gap)
• Implant does not migrate, change shape, or produce a foreign body reaction

Disadvantages

• Learning curve
• May extrude if ventricular mucosa is violated
• Requires "open" transcervical approach
• Unknown long-term effect

*Reprinted with permission. Adapted from Andrews et al.[1]

Table 7–6. Medialization laryngoplasty: complications and limitations.*

• Under-medialization secondary to intraoperative vocal fold edema
• Implant contamination from entry into the laryngeal ventricle
• Intracordal hematoma
• Transient stridor from postoperative edema
• Over-medialization of anterior 1/3 of the true vocal fold resulting in a strained voice
• Posterior glottic gap requiring addition of arytenoid adduction for closure
• Modest improvement with bilateral medialization for presbylaryngis

*Reprinted with permission. Adapted from Andrews et al.[1]

paralyzed vocal fold. Table 7–5 reviews the advantages and disadvantages of medialization laryngoplasty. Table 7–6 summarizes the complications and limitations of medialization laryngoplasty. Figure 7–1 shows the position of the vocal fold silastic implant.

Arytenoid Adduction

The goal of the **arytenoid adduction** procedure is to place traction on the muscular process of the arytenoid, mimicking the activity of the lateral cricoarytenoid muscle. The arytenoid is rotated internally, following an oblique axis, displacing the vocal process medially and caudally, thereby adducting the vocal fold. Additionally, the arytenoid, which may be subluxated anteriorly, may be pulled back to a more anatomic position. This corrects the vocal fold foreshortening and places the

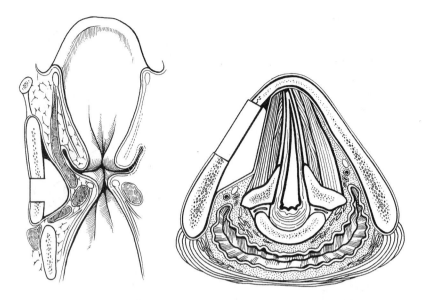

Figure 7–1. The implant should have smooth contours that gently displace the entire paraglottic space as needed. The maximum plane of medialization can be placed at any level, either within the window or below the level of the window, as determined by the depth gauge. Here, the maximum plant of medialization is at the lower border of the window, with the implant tapered posterior to the window to prevent contact with the muscular process of the arytenoid. Adapted from Andrews RJ, Netterville JL, Merati AL. In: Carrau RL, Murry T, eds. *Comprehensive Management of Swallowing Disorders.* San Diego, Calif: Singular Publishing Group; 1999:294.

affected vocal fold at the same level as the "functioning" fold, as shown in Figure 7–2.

Arytenoid adduction is designed specifically to close the posterior portion of the glottis in patients with unilateral paralysis of the vocal cord who have symptoms of significant glottic incompetence (breathy voice, aspiration, weak cough) and in whom flexible laryngoscopy reveals a unilateral laryngeal paralysis with a posterior gap during phonation. Factors that are associated with an increased risk of aspiration include a very wide glottal gap, deficits of the pharyngeal motor and sensory functions, and lack of relaxation of the cricopharyngeus muscle. This clinical scenario is frequently observed in patients with lesions of the proximal vagus nerve.

Arytenoid adduction is the only vocal fold medialization procedure that specifically addresses the posterior gap. This is achieved by rotating the arytenoid to achieve a favorable position of the vocal process and vocal fold, thus reducing the arytenoid subluxation.

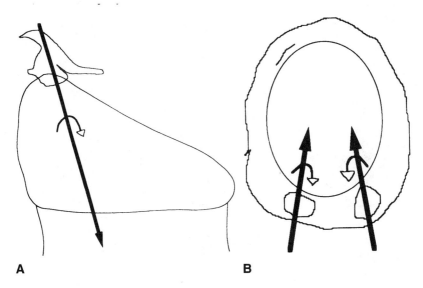

A   **B**

Figure 7–2. Axis of rotation in arytenoid adduction. From Newman TR, Hengesteg A, Lepage RP, Kaufman KR, Woodson GE. Three-dimensional motion of the arytenoid adduction procedure in cadaver larynges. *Ann Otol Rhinol Laryngol.* 1994;103:269, with permission. Adapted from Woodson GE. Chapter 42. Carrau RL, Murry T, eds. *Comprehensive Management of Swallowing Disorders.* San Diego, Calif: Singular Publishing Group; 1999:301.

CRICOPHARYNGEAL MYOTOMY

Cricopharyngeal myotomy should be considered for disorders in which there is incomplete upper esophageal sphincter segment relaxation or abnormal muscular contractions during the relaxation period. Patients with laryngeal paralysis due to pathology of the central nervous system or vagus nerve lesions frequently have associated impairment of pharyngeal motor and sensory function, which contribute to the swallowing impairment. In such patients, restoration of glottic closure may not be sufficient to correct the dysphagia and aspiration. In unilateral pharyngeal paresis, pharyngeal propulsion is often inadequate to propel the bolus past the cricopharyngeal sphincter, which, in cases with high vagal defects, may lose its ability to relax for the passage of the food bolus due to its bilateral innervation. This leads to pharyngeal "pooling" of the swallowed material and spillage over the arytenoids/aryepiglottic folds into the larynx (penetration). In the **insensate larynx,** it leads to **post-swallow aspiration.** In such patients,

Table 7–7. Cricopharyngeal myotomy.*

Indications

Dysphagia secondary to
• Central nervous system disorders
• Peripheral nervous system disorder
  Vagal injury (laryngeal/pharyngeal paralysis)
  Diabetic/peripheral neuropathy
• Muscular disease
  Oculopharyngeal dystrophy
  Steinert myotonic dystrophy
  Polymyositis
  Myasthenia gravis
• Hyperthyroidism/hypothyroidism
  Postsurgical
  Supraglottic laryngectomy
  Total laryngectomy
  Oral cavity/oropharyngeal resection
• Zenker's diverticulum
• Cricopharyngeal achalasia

Contraindications

• Severe weakness of the pharyngeal muscles (unable to propel bolus)
• Severe/uncontrolled GERD
• Pharyngeal varices
  Postbilateral neck dissections
  Thoracic outlet syndrome

*Adapted from Pou.[2]

Table 7–8. Cricopharyngeal myotomy: pitfalls and complications.*

Patient Factors/Poor Patient Selection

• Severe/uncontrolled GERD resulting in postoperative aspiration and pneumonia
• Extreme pharyngeal muscle weakness with inability to propel bolus

Surgical Errors

• Injury to the recurrent laryngeal nerve
• Accidental pharyngotomy
• Pharyngocutaneous fistula

*Adapted from Pou.[2]

cricopharyngeal myotomy is a useful adjunct to the vocal fold medialization. Table 7–7 presents the common indications for cricopharyngeal myotomy. Table 7–8 presents the pitfalls and complications of this procedure.

PALATOPEXY

Acquired **velopalatine incompetence** can result from partial or complete loss of the soft palate or neurogenic dysfunction of the soft palate. Neurogenic dysfunction resulting in either unilateral or bilateral paralysis of the soft palate creates varying degrees of velopalatine incompetence. During the process of swallowing, velopalatine incompetence is manifest by regurgitation of liquids, and rarely solids, into the nasopharynx with each swallow. Fifty percent of the patients with unilateral paralysis will improve over time, thus persisting with minimal complaints of swallowing dysfunction.

    Unilateral palatal adhesion (palatopexy) is indicated for patients with unilateral palatal paralysis. An adhesion is surgically created at the level of Passavant's ridge, a site of "normal" closure of the velopalatine valve. Even patients with very mild liquid reflux often have moderate to severe nasal quality to their speech, which dramatically improves with palatal adhesion. Figure 7–3 shows the adhesion location.

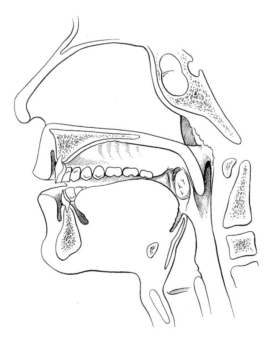

Figure 7–3. The adhesion is at the level of Pasavant's ridge to allow closure of the contralateral normal velopharynx. Adapted from Netterville JL. Chapter 44. In: Carrau RL, Murry T, eds. *Comprehensive Management of Swallowing Disorders.* San Diego, Calif: Singular Publishing Group; 1999:311.

SURGICAL CLOSURE OF THE LARYNX

Patients who continue to aspirate despite the use of conservative measures and adjunctive surgical procedures may require surgical closure of the larynx. The most common diagnoses of patients requiring a laryngotracheal separation are neurologic disorders such as cerebrovascular accidents (CVA) and amyotrophic lateral sclerosis (ALS). Laryngotracheal diversion, known as the standard Lindeman procedure, involves the creation of an anastomosis between the subglottic trachea and the esophagus and a permanent stoma from the distal trachea. With laryngotracheal separation (modified Lindeman procedure), the proximal subglottic trachea is closed as a blind pouch and a permanent stoma is created from the distal trachea, as shown in Figure 7–4. This technique of laryngotracheal separation best meets the desired criteria of simplicity, reliability, and reversibility, compared to other procedures shown in Table 7–9. Figure 7–5 outlines the scheme for treatment of patients with intractable aspiration.

Table 7–9. Surgical procedures used to separate esophagus from trachea.*

	Control of Aspiration	Preservation of Speech	Reversibility
Tracheostomy	−	+	+
Laryngeal stent	+/−	+/−	+
Laryngotracheal separation	+	−†	+
Total laryngectomy	+	−†	−

*Adapted from Snyderman.[3]
†Alaryngeal speech, either tracheoesophageal speech or esophageal speech, is possible.

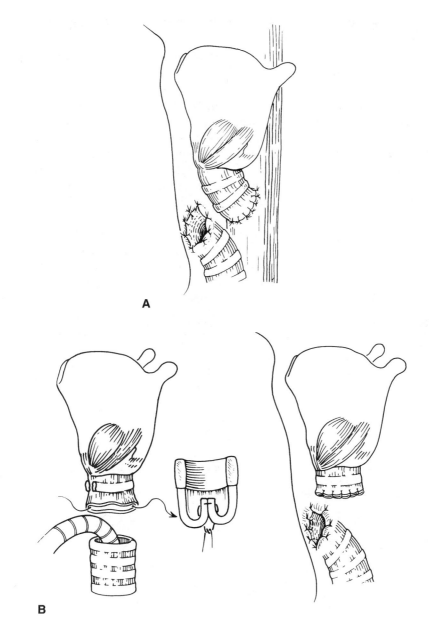

A

B

Figure 7–4. With laryngotracheal separation (modified Lindeman procedure), the proximal subglottic trachea is closed as a blind pouch and a permanent stoma is created from the distal trachea. Adapted from Snyderman CH. Chapter 45. In: Carrau RL, Murry T, eds. *Comprehensive Management of Swallowing Disorders.* San Diego, Calif: Singular Publishing Group; 1999:314.

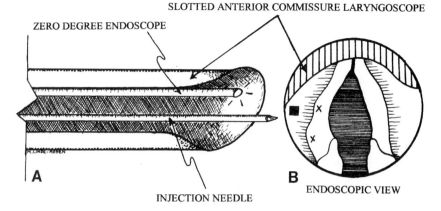

SLOTTED ANTERIOR COMMISSURE LARYNGOSCOPE

ZERO DEGREE ENDOSCOPE

A

INJECTION NEEDLE

B

ENDOSCOPIC VIEW

Figure 7–5. Schematic for treatment of patients with intractable aspiration. Asterisk indicates recurrent pneumonitis or hypoxia. From Current Opinion. In *Head Neck Surg.* 1994:2. Adapted from Rosen C. Chapter 40. In Carrau RL, Murry T, eds. *Comprehensive Management of Swallowing Disorders.* San Diego, Calif: Singular Publishing Group; 1999:315.

GASTROSTOMY

Percutaneous endoscopic gastrostomy (PEG) or open gastrostomy tubes provide an excellent route for feeding that can be temporary or permanent. These are discussed in Chapter 8. It should be noted, however, that the PEG does not necessarily prevent aspiration.

TRACHEOSTOMY

Tracheostomy implies the placement of a tube into the trachea through a transcervical incision. The most common indication for the procedure is the need for prolonged mechanical ventilation. Other factors influencing a recommendation for tracheostomy are shown in Table 7–10. A tracheostomy provides an airway and permits suctioning of the aspirated secretions. The presence of a tracheostomy does not enhance the ability of the patient to swallow and, in fact, will result in greater swallowing dysfunction and aspiration. Several maneuvers have been described to aid swallowing in patients with a tracheostomy, discussion of which follows.

Table 7–10. Factors influencing the recommendation for a tracheostomy in chronic ventilator-dependent patients.*

1. Need for prolonged mechanical ventilation
2. Primary diagnosis
3. Comorbidities
4. Nasal vs. oral tube
5. Patient comfort
6. Ease of endotracheal suction
7. Expected duration of ventilator support
8. Effect of reducing "dead space"
9. Patient motion
10. Complications of endotracheal tube
11. Perceived risk of laryngeal complications

*Adapted from Eibling and Carrau.[4]

Table 7–11. Expiratory valve advantages.*

• The patient can communicate verbally.
• Airflow provides proprioceptive cues during swallowing exercises and learning of maneuvers.
• True vocal fold adduction exercises will be maximized because of subglottic air pressure buildup.
• Improved pressure to aid in bolus propulsion.

*Adapted from Gross and Eibling.[5]

Expiratory Valve

An expiratory speaking valve is a removable valve that opens to permit inhalation but closes during expiration to divert the airflow through the larynx. The advantages of a speaking valve are shown in Table 7–11. The contraindications for the valve are shown in Table 7–12. It is important to monitor the patient when a speaking valve is first tried. Signs and symptoms of difficulty using a speaking valve are shown in Table 7–13.

Tracheostomy Tube—Fenestrated

A **fenestrated tracheostomy tube** is a tracheostomy tube with an opening to permit air to pass into the upper airway and oral cavity. Long-term use of this tube is ill-advised, as the friction of the fenestra

Table 7–12. Contraindications to the use of a speaking valve.*

- Unconscious/comatose patients
- Behavior problems
- Medical instability, especially pulmonary failure
- Tracheal stenosis
- Airway obstruction above the tube that precludes expiration through the glottis
- Thick and copious secretions that persist after valve placement
- Foam-filled tracheotomy tube cuff
- Total laryngectomy or laryngotracheal separation
- Insufficient passage for air around the tube, either with the cuff down or with a cuffless tube
- Inability to maintain adequate ventilation with cuff deflation in ventilator-dependent patient
- Patients with cognitive disorders

*Adapted from Gross and Eibling.[5]

Table 7–13. Signs and symptoms of difficulty tolerating the valve.*

- Increasing respiratory rate over time with or without nasal flaring, head bobbing
- Increased irritability and/or restlessness, or fear and anxiety
- Decreased chest movement
- Skin color changes such as pallor, cyanosis, mottling

*Adapted from Gross and Eibling.[5]

against the tracheal walls produces exuberant granulation tissue, which has been associated with bleeding and/or life-threatening airway compromise.

Decannulation

The patient's ability to tolerate **decannulation** can be estimated by the amount of oral and tracheal secretions and by the patient's tolerance of tube capping. Decannulation is the most effective single intervention to enhance swallowing in patients with a tracheostomy.

Cricothyrotomy

Cricothyrotomy consists of an incision through the skin and the cricothyroid membrane for relief of respiratory obstruction. It is used in lieu of tracheostomy in emergency situations and electively in selected patients undergoing surgery that requires a median sternotomy (e.g., cardiac bypass surgery).

REFERENCES

1. Andrews RJ, Netterville JL, Merati AL. In: Carrau RL, Murry T, eds. *Comprehensive Management of Swallowing Disorders.* San Diego, Calif: Singular Publishing Group; 1999:291–294.
2. Pou A. In: Carrau RL, Murry T, eds. *Comprehensive Management of Swallowing Disorders.* San Diego, Calif: Singular Publishing Group; 1999:306, 308.
3. Snyderman CH. In: Carrau RL, Murry T, eds. *Comprehensive Management of Swallowing Disorders.* San Diego, Calif: Singular Publishing Group; 1999:315.
4. Eibling DE, Carrau RL. In: Carrau RL, Murry T, eds. *Comprehensive Management of Swallowing Disorders.* San Diego, Calif: Singular Publishing Group; 1999:260.
5. Gross RD, Eibling DE. In: Carrau RL, Murry T, eds. *Comprehensive Management of Swallowing Disorders.* San Diego, Calif: Singular Publishing Group; 1999:255, 258.

CHAPTER

8

Nutrition and Diets

INTRODUCTION

The importance of proper nutrition cannot be overestimated in the management of dysphagia. Nutritional status can have a significant impact on rehabilitation, especially affecting those factors related to self-esteem, psychosocial aspects, and overall quality of life. The management of dysphagia not only requires the treatment team to ensure the safety of swallowing but also requires the team to ensure that the patient is adequately nourished in amount of calories, content of calories, and essential nutrients. Failure to achieve proper nourishment will result in **malnutrition,** another obstacle in the recovery process.

Proper nutrition can be achieved through oral or non-oral diets or from a combination of the two. In the recovery process from surgery and/or radiation therapy for cancer of the head and neck, nutrition usually begins with a non-oral diet, often through a nasogastric tube, and then proceeds to a combined oral–non-oral diet and finally an oral diet in most cases. Stroke recovery is similar; however, with the stroke patient, the patient's cognitive status, degree of alertness, and understanding of the rehabilitation process must also be taken into account. In some cases, a period of enteral feeding may be necessary.

A comprehensive dysphagia treatment program makes extensive use of the **nutritionist** in order to prevent malnutrition, maintain or increase muscle mass, and maintain an adequate immune status. The

Table 8–1. Components of a nutritional assessment.*

Physical Exam

- Muscle and fat stores
- Coordination skills
- Presence of decubitus
- Skin turgor
- Ascites
- Feeding skills
- Dentition
- Edema
- Anthropometrics

Medical History

- Recent surgical history
- History of medical comorbidity
- Gastrointestinal history
- Review swallowing function
- Alterations of gastrointestinal tract
- Planned medical procedures
- Neuromuscular conditions
- Cognitive status

Nutritional History

- Diet history
- Food intolerances or aversions
- Complaints of anorexia
- Use of vitamin supplements
- History of pica eating
- Previous or current diet modifications
- Use of nutritional supplements
- Normal eating patterns
- Alcohol intake
- Ability to use utensils

Medication Review

- Drug/nutrient interactions
- Administration schedule
- Impact on feeding schedule and ability to eat and cognitive status

Biochemical Data

- Visceral protein store measures (albumin, transferrin, prealbumin)
- Electrolytes
- Glucose
- BUN/creatinine
- Hemoglobin/hematocrit
- Total lymphocyte count

*From Molseed.[1]

nutritionist may elect to perform a comprehensive nutrition assessment, as seen in Table 8–1, or may limit the assessment to the specific needs of the patient at various stages for which the treatment is being modified. The nutritionist works closely with the speech and language pathologist and other rehabilitation team members to select foods or supplements for oral feeding that provide proper nourishment while at the same time maximize proper oral control, transit, and timing of swallowing. If the feeding is non-oral, the nutritionist monitors the selection, amount, and timing of the enteral feeding to assure proper protein-caloric requirements.

In this chapter, the characteristics of liquids and foods are examined in relationship to the safety and nutrition for the dysphagic patient. Oral diets and non-oral feeding alternatives are reviewed. Malnutrition and its consequences as it relates to dysphagia are considered. Nutrition and its importance in the recovery from sickness, injury, or surgery are extensive topics and have far-reaching implications. Comprehensive reviews of nutrition including enteral feeding requirements, calorie intake calculation, and nutritional content may be found in publications by the American Dietetic Association.[2,3]

PROPERTIES OF LIQUIDS AND FOODS

The study of fluids and their properties has influenced the development of thickeners to change the property of a liquid or food substance so that it may be used in the diet of a dysphagic patient. This field of study is known as **rheology.** It has provided a basis for developing some degree of consistency in nutrition. To this date, standards have not been established but clinical terminology is now becoming more common. Fluids can now be assessed for their properties through rheology and its analysis. To understand **rheologic analysis** completely goes beyond the scope of most members of the dysphagia team. However, a basic knowledge in rheology and how it relates to normal and disordered swallowing is important to the clinician.

Terminology

Although its clinical significance is still largely undetermined, the rheological properties of foods and fluids may be useful for the study and development of standard dysphagia diets and feeding protocols. More importantly, by obtaining standard foods and/or liquids, instrumental testing—whether it be a modified barium swallow, fiberoptic endoscopic evaluation of swallowing, or other—can also approach standardization.

The most common terms relating to the study of fluid-flow properties are the following:

▶ **Constitutive equation:** An equation relating to stress with strain and sometimes other variables including time, temperature, and concentration.

▶ **Creep test:** A test to determine the deformation of a material exposed to a constant stress. These are like relaxation tests, but a constant stress is applied rather than a constant strain. The simplest creep test would be to apply a weight on top of a sample and record the change in shape (strain) over time; for example, placing an orange on a bowl of pudding and measuring the deformation over time.

- **Density:** The compactness of a substance; the ratio of its mass to its volume measured in grams per milliliter (g/ml or kg/ml).
- **Homogeneous:** Well mixed and compositionally similar regardless of location.
- **Incompressible:** Material that shows no change in density when a constant stress is applied (e.g., water).
- **Isotropic:** The material response is not a function of location or direction.
- ▶ **Kinematic viscosity:** Viscosity divided by the density of the material.
- **Laminar flow:** Nonturbulent flow.
- **Linear viscoelasticity:** Viscoelasticity within the region where stress and strain are linearly related.
- ▶ **Newtonian fluid:** A fluid with a linear relationship between shear stress and shear rate with a yield stress. The viscosity of a Newtonian fluid does not vary with shear rate.
- ▶ **Non-Newtonian fluid:** Any fluid deviating from Newtonian behavior. Fluids that are suspensions. The attractive force between suspensioned particles weakens as shear rate increases.
- **Rheogram:** A graph showing rheological relationships.
- ▶ **Rheology:** The study of properties of fluids. Rheological models are mathematical expressions providing a "flow fingerprint" for fluid foods.
- ▶ **Rheometer:** An instrument used for measuring rheological properties. This device is used in creep tests.
- ▶ **Shear (strain) rate:** Change in strain with respect to time.
- ▶ **Strain:** Relative deformation.
- ▶ **Viscoelastic:** A material having both viscous and elastic properties.
- ▶ **Viscometer:** A device used to measure the resistance of a material to flowing.
- ▶ **Viscosity:** Resistance to flow or alteration of shape by a substance as a result of molecular cohesion. Newton's postulate reasons that if the shear stress is doubled, the velocity gradient (shear strain rate) within the fluid is doubled. For fluids, strain is measured in terms of shear rate, and the shear stress may be expressed as some function of shear rate and viscosity. For **Newtonian fluids,** the viscosity function is constant and called the coefficient of viscosity or **Newtonian viscosity.**

Applications of Rheology

Viscosity is a prime variable in the study of **Newtonian fluids.** For simplicity, the clinician may view the **viscosity** of a fluid as being proportional to the force required to move it through an area. A bolus that is twice as viscous requires roughly twice as much power from the swallow musculature to transport the bolus.[4] Viscosity sheer rate profiles are shown in Table 8–2. As can be seen, standard barium is a **non-Newtonian fluid** with a density greater than thin barium or a cordial fluid. Thus, when studying swallow patterns with the modified barium swallow, the clinician should note the type and consistency of the barium. Where regular modified barium swallow studies are done, premixed barium consistencies should be available to the clinician so that when a report is generated, the treatment team will know the conditions under which the patient was evaluated.

The instrumental assessment of swallowing provides an indication of acceptable viscosities for maximum safe swallowing. It is important that the entire team understands the viscosities and uses consistent mixtures during the treatment. Table 8–3 lists common

Table 8–2. Viscosity shear rate profiles and density measurements of various fluids.*

Fluid	Newtonian or Non-Newtonian	Density (kg/m)	Viscosity Range
Fluid 1: thin cordial	Newtonian	980	Constant cP = 2cP
Fluid 2: thickened cordial	Non-Newtonian	1,000	Range of cP 100,000–300 cP from 1 to 100 1/s, "shear thinning"
Fluid 3: standard barium (nectar)	Non-Newtonian	2,800	Range of cP 4,000–200 cP from 1 to 100 1/s, "shear thinning + plateau"
Fluid 4: thin barium	Newtonian	2,300	Constant cP = 26 cP, "poor resolution at low rates"
Fluid 5: thickened barium	Non-Newtonian	2,500	Range of cP 30,000–900 cP, from 1–100 1/s "shear thinning"

*From Cichero et al.[5]

Table 8–3. Materials used to adjust the consistency of the bolus.

Thinning Agents/Blenderizing Agents

• Milk
• Juice
• Gravy
• Tomato juice

Thickening Agents

• Cornstarch
• Baby cereal (or other dehydrated baby food)
• Mashed potato flakes
• Instant pudding
• Unflavored gelatin

*Adapted from Molseed.[1]

agents that may be used to alter the viscosity of fluids. Ideally, these agents should be mixed with predetermined amounts of barium to provide consistent references to the dysphagia treatment. Eventually, commercial products listing the density and perhaps the coefficient of viscosity for test and treatment materials will be available.

Solid Texture

The goal of treatment for swallowing disorders is oral intake of all foods, liquids as well as solids. The intake of solid foods is related to the severity of impairment, adequate dentition and muscular strength for chewing, and coordination for bolus transit and control.

The modification of oral feeding requires an understanding of liquid viscosities and food textures. **Texture** refers to the composition of food. Common texture terminology includes **nectar, puree, sticky, mechanical soft,** and so on. These terms are purely perceptual in nature as even common terms such as puree or nectar can have a wide range of viscosities and densities. Table 8–4 summarizes the common clinical terms for textures, ranging from thin liquids to foods requiring mastication. The table provides examples of each texture and their properties along the viscosity continuum.

Table 8–5 provides a correlation of the textures with the severity of the swallowing disorder. Since the terms are somewhat general, the clinician must be aware of the instrumental test results, the medical history, and the cognitive status of the patient when interpreting impairment level and food texture. The assessment process would benefit from the examiner using consistent test amounts and consistent mixtures. Thus, even though there may not be consistency between or among institutions, tests done at the same institution may have internal consistency.

ORAL NUTRITION AND DYSPHAGIA DIETS

Oral nutrition is the goal for most patients presenting with dysphagia due to stroke or for those after receiving head and neck cancer surgery. Conversely, for patients with progressive neuromuscular diseases, oral nutrition may be the starting level of intervention and this may downgrade to enteral nutrition as their primary disease advances.

Oral diets are organized on the basis of viscosity of the foods and liquids. Safe swallowing requires temporal management of the neuromuscular behaviors at each stage of the swallow.

Dysphagia Diets

Dysphagia diets vary considerably from facility to facility. Attempts to develop standard dysphagia diets are underway. Although there are no standards at present, all dysphagia diets should adjust food/liquid intake for (1) amount, (2) consistency, and (3) timing of the meal to achieve maximal nutrition with minimal swallowing difficulty. Oral dysphagia diets are typically a stepwise progression of bolus consistencies and may be grouped into four levels:

▶ **Level 1:** Pureed food and thickened liquid—the most conservative level. This diet is used in patients with severe oral preparatory, oral phase, and pharyngeal dysphagia.
▶ **Level 2:** Pureed and mechanically altered foods, plus thick or thickened liquids and very soft foods that require minimal chewing (e.g., cottage cheese, macaroni, pancake with syrup). This diet is used in patients with deficits of the oral phase or with decreased pharyngeal peristalsis. This diet is also the most common diet for those patients who are suspected or identified to suffer aspiration. It is first used under therapeutic control, and then the patient is advanced to use it without monitoring when the clinician deems it safe to do so.
▶ **Level 3:** Mechanically altered and soft foods with liquids allowed as tolerated. This diet is advised for individuals who are beginning to chew and to rehabilitate chewing and bolus propulsion.
▶ **Level 4:** Soft foods and all liquids, avoiding rough or coarse foods. This diet usually precedes advancement to regular diet.

Table 8–4. Continuum of textures or viscosities (modified from Susan McKenzie, M.S., and Beverly Lorens, R.D., M.S.).*

	Thin Liquids	Thick Liquids	Slippery Puree
E X A M P L E	Assumed to be at body temperature: apple juice; cranberry juice; non, low-fat, and whole milk; fruit ice; sherbet; jello; soft drinks.	Assumed to be at body temperature: tomato juice, nectar, apple juice with thickener, instant breakfast, ≥ 1.5 cal/cc commercial supplement.	Assumed to be at body temperature: pudding, custard, puree fruit, puree vegetables (not starches).
P R O P E R T I E S	Easily deformed, moves very readily in response to gravity and compression.	Less easily deformed than thin liquids, moves fairly readily in response to gravity or compression.	Less easily deformed, so may obstruct a narrow passage. Slides in response to gravity or compression.

*From Leonard and Kendall.[6]

Consistency Modifications

▶ **Liquid modification:** Used to increase or decrease the viscosity of the liquid in order to achieve bolus control.
Thin: Clear liquids, milk, coffee and tea, and broth based soups.
Thick: Milkshakes, strained cream soups, nectars.
Thickened: Thin or thick liquids may require thickening agents to assure the appropriate consistency. Table 8–6 lists commercial thickening agents. The amounts to be mixed will vary substantially, and the clinician may resort to a "trial and error" mixture consistency for each individual.

▶ **Solid food modification:** A means to advancing the diet in steps consistent with patient progress.

▶ **Pureed/liquefied:** Regular food may be blenderized with added liquid as needed to form a smooth consistency. The consistency may vary from a thick liquid consistency to a paste-like consistency. The consistency of baby food is often best tolerated; however, it should be adjusted to meet the individual's needs.

Table 8–4. *continued*

	Puree	Foods Requiring Mastication (in Order of Ascending Difficulty)		
E X A M P L E	Mashed potatoes, puree scrambled eggs, puree meat.	Ground meat, regular scrambled eggs, canned fruit, soft cooked carrots, beets, bread.	Chopped meat, sandwiches (tuna, egg, bologna).	Unrestricted diet.
P R O P E R T I E S	Less easily deformed, thus can obstruct narrow passage. Transferred mostly by compression.	As the bolus becomes more viscous, it is less and less easily deformed, less likely to move in response to gravity, more reliant on dental and lingual competence for mastication and transit, sensory competence and judgment of bolus characteristics, adequate salivation, and healthy mucosa.		

▶ **Mechanically altered:** Chopped and ground foods, very soft foods such as pasta and casseroles, and foods that easily form a cohesive bolus are included in this diet.

▶ **Soft:** Naturally soft foods that require a minimal amount of chewing are found on this diet. Meat may need to be cut in small pieces and rough food such as nuts, popcorn, raw vegetables and salads are avoided. Avoid foods that crumble or that are of mixed consistency.

See Table 8–7 for three categories of foods that are not well tolerated by individuals with swallowing problems.

NON-ORAL DIETS

A large number of patients are unable to take adequate nutrition orally. This may be temporary in patients who have had surgery for oral, pharyngeal, or laryngeal disease; patients who are acutely recovering from

Table 8–5. Solid texture: correlation with swallowing severity.*

	NPO†	Pureed
Functional Impairment Level	Severe impairment: all nourishment via alternate feeding method (NPO); trial oral intake with SLP only.	Moderately severe impairment: alternate feeding method is primary source of nourishment. Limited, inconsistent success with oral intake. Requires constant supervision; some assistance required in feeding but SLP introduces new items or techniques.
Dysphagia Severity Rating: Parkinson's Disease	Severe dysphagia: more than 10% aspiration for all consistencies. "Nothing by mouth" recommended.	Moderate severe dysphagia: patient aspirates 5% to 10% on one or more consistencies, with potential for aspiration of all consistencies. Potential for aspiration minimized by use of specific swallowing instructions. Cough reflex absent or nonprotective. Alternative mode of feeding required to maintain patient's nutritional need. If pulmonary status is compromised, "NPO" may be indicated.
Severity Scale Primarily related to ALS	Aspiration of secretions: secretions cannot be managed noninvasively. Patient rarely swallows. Secretions are managed with suction/medication: patient cannot safely manage any PO intake. Patient usually swallows reflexively.	Tube feeding with occasional PO nutrition. Primary nutrition and hydration are accomplished by tube. Patient receives less than 50% of nutrition. PO intake alone is no longer adequate. Patient uses or needs a tube to supplement intake. Patient continues to take significant (less than 50%) PO. Liquified diet: oral PO intake is adequate. Nutrition is limited primarily to liquified diet. Adequate thin liquid intake usually a problem. Patient may force self to eat.

*Adapted from Cherney et al[7]
†Key: NPO = Nothing by mouth

SLP = speech and language pathologist
PO = oral intake

Table 8–5. *continued*

Mechanically Altered	Advanced	Regular
Mid-moderate impairment: fairly reliable swallowing of prescribed diet but may have difficulty with clear liquids or solids; requires supervision.	Mild impairment: intake of regular diet with some food restrictions; may require specific techniques or procedures to achieve successful swallowing. Does not require close supervision.	Minimal impairment: efficient chewing and swallowing of all food consistencies with occasional episodes of coughing and/or requires additional time for adequate intake. Normal: safe and efficient chewing and swallowing of all food consistencies.
Mild-moderate dysphagia: potential for aspiration exists but is diminished by specific swallowing techniques and a modified diet. Time required for eating is significantly increased, and supplemental nutrition may be indicated.	Mild dysphagia: oral pharyngeal dysphagia is present but can be managed by specific swallowing suggestions. Slight modification in consistency of diet may be indicated.	Minimal dysphagia: videofluoroscopy shows slight deviance from a normal swallow. Patient may report a change in sensation during swallow. No change in diet is required. Normal swallowing mechanism.
Soft diet: diet is limited primarily to soft foods. Requires some special meal preparation Prolonged time or small bite size: mealtime has significantly lengthened and smaller bite sizes are necessary. Patient must concentrate on swallowing liquids.	Minor swallowing problems: complains of some swallowing difficulties. Maintains an essentially regular diet. Isolated choking episodes. Normal abnormalities: only patient notices slight indicator such as food lodging in the recesses of the mouth or sticking in the throat.	Normal swallowing: patient denies any difficulty chewing or swallowing. Examination demonstrates no abnormality.

Table 8–6. Thickeners: products and producers.*

Thick-it™ **Thick-it 2™**	Milani Foods, Inc. Does not sell directly to consumer but often can be ordered by local pharmacy. Thick-it 2™ is more expensive than Thick-it™, but less is needed. Thick-it 2™ should be mixed in a blender for smoother results.
Nutrathik™ **Thicken Right™** **Puree Shape and Serve™**	Menu Magic Foods, Division of Diamond Crystal Specialty Foods; Corporate Office, Wilmington, Mass. Laura Cooper, Marketing Manager, (800) 225-0592. Nutrathik™ 20 cals/tbs, fortified with vitamins and minerals. Thicken Right™ 15 cal/tbs. Puree Shape & Serve™ 20 cals/tbs, provides shape and texture to meats and vegetables.
Thick and Easy™	Contact: American Pharmacy (800) 692-7293. Shipping by UPS.
Thicken-Up™ **Puree Appeal™**	Delmark-Sandoz Nutrition. May purchase through TAD Enterprises, 9356 Pleasant, Tinley Park, Ill 60477; (800)438-6153. 8 oz can contains 51 tbs. Also available are thickened juices and a product to add to pureed foods. Puree Appeal™ contains 30 cals/tbs.
Thixx™ **Super Thixx™** **Ultra Thixx™** **Vitamin Fortified** **Ultra Thixx™**	Bernard Foods, Consumer Products Division, (800)325-5409, catalog. For consumer orders: The Diet Shoppe, Calco Company, 3540 W. Jarvis Avenue, Skokie, Ill 60076; (800)325-5409. Thixx™ mixes easily with hot or cold beverages, 16 cal/tbs. An 8 oz can contains 335 tbs. Reportedly, Thixx™ works better in hot products. Super Thixx™, 24 cal/tbs. Has twice the thickening strength of Thixx™. It is especially formulated for use in blenders. An 11 oz can contains 52 tbs.

*Adapted from Leonard and Kendall[6]

Table 8–7. Foods and consistencies not tolerated by individuals with dysphagia.*

Crumbly and Noncohesive Foods

- Plain ground meat, chicken, or fish
- Scrambled eggs
- Rice
- Jello
- Crackers

- Peas, corn, or legumes
- Cornbread
- Cottage cheese
- Coconut
- Nuts and seeds

Mixed-Consistency Foods

- Vegetable soup
- Soup with large pieces or chunks of food
- Cold cereal with milk
- Citrus fruit

- Salad with dressing
- Canned fruit
- Gelatin with fruit
- Yogurt with fruit

Sticky Foods

- Dry mashed potatoes
- Peanut butter
- Fresh white or refined wheat bread
- Fudge or butterscotch sauce/caramel
- Bagels or soft rolls

*Adapted from Keenan.[8]

a stroke; or those patients with a neuromuscular degenerative disorder who no longer can tolerate oral nutrition.

Enteral feeding is that type of feeding that occurs by way of the intestinal tract. In patients who are unable to take adequate nutrition by mouth but otherwise have a functioning gastrointestinal (GI) tract (i.e., stomach and intestinal tract), enteral feeding is the best alternative to maintain nutrition and to avoid dehydration and malnutrition. Enteral routes include three main pathways: (1) **nasoenteric** (nasogastric or nasoduodenal); (2) **jejunostomy** (entering in the jejunum, the small intestine between the duodenum and the ileum); and (3) **gastrostomy** (entering into the stomach). A **gastrojejunostomy** is a tube that enters through the stomach but the tip is advanced to the jejunum. Table 8–8 summarizes the common feeding tubes with their advantages and disadvantages.

Table 8–8. Feeding tubes: types, advantages, and disadvantages.*

Access Site	Advantages
Nasogastric	• Minimally invasive, easy placement • Suitable for short-term use • Transitional to bolus feeding • Radiographic confirmation not necessarily required but recommended for liability issues
Nasoduodenal	• Minimally invasive, easy placement • Suitable for short-term use • Reduced risk of pulmonary aspiration • Useful in conditions of gastroparesis or impaired stomach emptying • Useful if esophageal reflux present • Allows for feeding when bowel sounds are diminished or absent
Nasojejunal	• Same advantages as nasoduodenal • Placement of tip further down GI tract minimizes dislocation to stomach • 60″ length tubes available offering even greater placement security
Cervical esophagostomy	• Improved cosmetic appeal as end of tube more easily concealed • Ease of feeding over gastrostomy as do not need to undress • More suitable for long-term feeding
Gastrostomy	• Suitable for long-term feeding • Cosmetically more appealing than a nasally placed tube • Minimizes risk of tube migration and aspiration due to voluntary or accidental dislocation of nasoenteric tube by patient • Percutaneous placement available (PEG)[†] • Some GT[†] have large bore tubes that minimize occlusion from medications and high viscosity formulas • Most suitable of all tubes for use of homemade formula, provided tip is placed in stomach and it is a large bore tube • Bolus feeding option available if tip of tube in stomach
Jejunostomy	• Suitable for long-term feeding • Minimizes risk of aspiration • Positive gag reflex need not be present • Useful if esophageal reflux is present • Does not depend on functioning stomach • Percutaneous placement (PEJ)[†]

*Adapted and modified from Gottschlich et al[9] and from Leonard and Kendall.[6]
[†]Key: PEG = percutaneous endoscopic gastrostomy

Table 8–8. *continued*

Disadvantages

- Cosmetic feeding tube visible unless patient self-inserts each feeding
- Risk of sinusitis
- Lack of intact gag reflex may (not necessarily) indicate increased aspiration risk
- Stomach must be uninvolved with primary disease

- Requires radiographic confirmation of placement
- Cosmetic: feeding tube is visible

- Requires 43″ length feeding tube
- May not remain placed in duodenum due to tube migration
- Typically, smaller diameter tube than NG, more prone to plugging if not properly maintained

- Similar disadvantages as nasoduodenal, except placement of tip more secure

- Although more suitable for long-term feeding, the lower esophageal sphincter is stented open and same concerns for gastric and esophageal reflux with possible pulmonary aspiration are present as with the NG feeding tube

- Potential risk of pulmonary aspiration
- Lack of intact gag reflex and/or presence of esophageal reflux may indicate increased risk of aspiration
- Insertion site care needed
- Potential skin excoriation at stoma site from leakage of gastric secretion
- Potential fistula at insertion site after GT removal
- If GT feeding tip port is placed in duodenum, usually a smaller bore tube is used and it is subject to more occlusion risk

- Typically smaller bore tubes than a GT and risk of occlusion from medication or viscous formula
- Stoma care needed
- Potential skin excoriation at stoma site from leakage of gastric secretions
- Bolus feeding not an option
- Potential fistula at stoma site after JT removal

GT = gastrostomy tube
PEJ = percutaneous endoscopic jejunostomy

Nasogastric and Nasoduodenal Tubes

Nasogastric tubes (NG tubes) are the most commonly placed tubes. An NG tube is typically placed with the expectation that swallow rehabilitation will be aggressive and short-term (3 to 21 days). In some cases, the NG tube must be replaced by a more permanent feeding tube, often needed as the result of additional morbidity that was not expected at the time of the initial NG tube placement.

Nasoduodenal tubes are also used for short-term dysphagia. They are useful when there is a strong suspicion of **esophageal reflux** or **gastroparesis** (inability to empty the stomach due either to bilateral vagotomy or neural damage to the vagus nerve). Gastroparesis is often found in patients with diabetes mellitus.

Gastrostomy Tubes

A **gastrostomy tube** is surgically placed directly into the stomach. Feedings per gastric tube can be administered by continuous feeding or by bolus feed. Gastrostomy tubes are preferred for long-term, non-oral feeding because they are less likely to become dislodged than nasal tubes. For the patient who is ambulatory, gastrostomy tubes are easily hidden, avoiding social embarrassment. In addition, medications are more easily administered than through a nasogastric tube due to the large bore of the gastrostomy tube. Gastrostomy tubes are less likely to clog than NG tubes, and they do not irritate the interarytenoid area.

A gastrostomy can be created through a **percutaneous endoscopic** (PEG) route or by transabdominal (i.e., laparotomy or laparoscopic) placement of a tube or creation of a stoma. The PEG has become the procedure of choice since it can be done in the intensive care unit or the procedure room under local anesthesia and sedation. In general, the PEG takes less time and costs less than laparoscopic assisted or open gastrostomies, although the tube placed is smaller than the one placed with the other techniques.

Anatomically, the gastrostomy can be classified as those that are lined with serosa (temporary) and those lined by mucosa (permanent). Functionally, this relates not only to the care of the gastrostomy site but also to the procedures that are required for reversal when no longer needed. Serosa-lined gastrostomies include PEG, laparoscopic assisted gastrostomy, and some open (Stamm) gastrostomy. They are, in fact, serosa-lined gastrocutaneous fistulas. The lining of the tract is granulation tissue, which will quickly close if the tube is removed for any reason. Therefore, if this type of gastric tube is displaced, it must be replaced within the 4 to 6 hours that the tract will remain open.

The following problems are the most commonly encountered associated with placement of a gastrostomy tube:

▶ Excoriated skin around gastrostomy site
▶ Cellulitis around gastrostomy site
▶ Abscess at gastrostomy site (rare)
▶ Catheter clogging
▶ Gastrostomy tube extrusion

A "permanent" or mucosa-lined gastrostomy (e.g., Janeway gastrostomy) requires a laparotomy in the operating room and is constructed by creating a tube of stomach, which is brought out through the anterior abdominal wall. The mucosa-lined gastrocutaneous fistula, as opposed to the serosa-lined fistula, will not close if the feeding tube is removed.

The decision to opt for non-oral feeding is often a critical one for the patient and family. Instrumental testing may provide the basis for the decision, but the decision is not based solely on radiographic, manometric, or endoscopic assessment. Other factors used to decide in favor of non-oral feeding include (1) time required to swallow, (2) energy level of patient, (3) need for alternative route for medications, (4) repeated episodes of dehydration, (5) unexplained weight loss or signs of malnutrition, and (6) repeated signs of aspiration. All of the issues, those related to diagnostic findings as well as the clinical observations, must be discussed with the patient and family members when the option for non-oral feeding is part of the treatment plan.

It is equally important to present a strong rationale for the recommendation of non-oral feedings in a patient with a progressive neuromuscular disease such as amyotrophic lateral sclerosis (ALS). Logemann[10] has pointed out that the time to complete one swallow has diagnostic significance. This factor along with others already noted should be considered when a feeding tube is planned. The patient with ALS and other patients with neuromuscular degeneration will only benefit from a feeding tube when they still have the energy and desire to maintain their nutrition. Waiting until the patient is near the end of life denies him or her of the quality of life that might otherwise remain if nutrition is maintained.

MALNUTRITION AND DEHYDRATION

Patients with swallowing disorders should be monitored for signs of malnutrition and dehydration. The nutritionist regularly reviews body weight, caloric intake, liquid intake, feeding schedules (oral and non-oral), medication/nutrition interactions, and biochemical data. However, it is up to the entire dysphagia team to be alert for those factors that lead to dehydration and malnutrition.

Stroke patients are the largest group of individuals with dysphagia to be at risk for malnutrition and dehydration. Cognitive defects, hemiparesis, spatial neglect, and motor disabilities all contribute to the risk of malnutrition in stroke patients. Malnutrition in stroke patients may be as high as 56% during some point of a 3-week hospital stay.[11]

Malnutrition can occur as a result of poor or inadequate oral or non-oral intake. **Protein-calorie malnutrition** (PCM) is one of the most common types of malnutrition and has the power to fatigue muscles, alter the neuromuscular function of the swallow muscles, and contribute to increasing the severity of dysphagia. Other factors such as stress reaction, respiratory and urinary infections, and bedsores may develop or increase once malnutrition is present. Given these comorbidity factors, one might expect longer hospital stays, poorer outcome, and greater risk of further illness with the presence of malnutrition.

When there is a concern about malnutrition, weight, and weight history, serum albumin and prealbumin are capable of identifying the majority of patients requiring nutritional attention. In the acute and rehabilitation setting, weight would be checked every 2 days. For home health care, weight should be checked at every visit.

REFERENCES

1. Molseed L. Clinical evaluation of swallowing: the nutritionist's perspective. In: Carrau RL, Murry T, eds. *Comprehensive Management of Swallowing Disorders.* San Diego, Calif: Singular Publishing Group; 1999:60,239.
2. Nutrition management in dysphagia. In: *Manual of Clinical Dietetics.* 5th ed. Chicago: American Dietetic Association; 1996.
3. Lewis MM, Kidder JA. *Nutrition Practice Guidelines for Dysphagia.* Chicago: American Dietetic Association; 1996.
4. Li M, Brasseur JG, Kern MK, Dodds WJ. Viscosity measurements of barium sulfate mixtures for use in motility studies of the pharynx and esophagus. *Dysphagia.* 1992;7:17–30.
5. Cichero JA, Hay G, Murdoch BE, Halley M. Videofluoroscopic fluids versus mealtime fluids: differences in viscosity and density made clear. *J Med Speech Lang Path.* 1997;5:210.
6. Leonard R, Kendall K. *Dysphagia Assessment and Treatment Planning.* San Diego, Calif: Singular Publishing Group; 1997:240–241, 250–251.

7. Cherney LR, Pannell JJ, Cantieri CA. Clinical evaluation of dysphagia in adults. In: Cherney LR, ed. *Clinical Management of Dysphagia in Adults and Children*. Gaithersburg, Md: Aspen Publishers; 1994.

8. Keenan RJ. In: Carrau RL, Murry T, eds. *Comprehensive Management of Swallowing Disorders*. San Diego, Calif: Singular Publishing Group; 1999:238–239.

9. Gottschlich M, Matarese L, Shronts E. *Nutrition Supports Dietetics Core Curriculum*. 2nd ed. American Society for Parenteral and Enteral Nutrition; 1998.

10. Logemann JA. Factors affecting ability to resume oral nutrition in the oropharyngeal dysphagic individual. *Dysphagia*. 1990; 4:202–208.

11. Axelsson K, Asplund K, Norberg A, Ericsson S. Eating problems and nutritional status during hospital stay of patients with severe stroke. *J Am Diet Assoc*. 1989;89:1092–1096.

References

Peer-Reviewed References

Alberts MJ, Horner J, Gray L, Brazer SR. Aspiration after stroke: lesion analysis by brain MRI. *Dysphagia*. 1992;7:170–173.

Ali GN, Laundl TM, Wallace KL, deCarle DJ, Cook IJS. Influence of cold stimulation on the normal pharyngeal swallow response. *Dysphagia*. 1996;11:2–8.

Ali GN, Wallace KL, Laundl TM, Hunt DR, deCarle DJ, Cook IJ. Predictors of outcome following cricopharyngeal disruption for pharyngeal dysphagia. *Dysphagia*. 1997;12:133–139.

Anselmino M, Zaninotto G, Costantini M, et al. Esophageal motor function in primary Sjögren's syndrome: correlation with dysphagia and xerostomia. *Dig Dis Sci*. 1997;42:113–118.

Ardran G, Kemp F. Some important factors in the assessment of oropharyngeal function. *Dev Med Child Neurol*. 1970;12:158–166.

Arvedson JC, Rogers BT. Pediatric swallowing and feeding disorder. *J Med Speech Lang Pathol*. 1993;1:203–221.

Aviv JE. Sensory discrimination in the larynx and hypopharynx. *Otolaryngol Head Neck Surg*. 1997;116:331–334.

Aviv JE, Sacco RL, Mohr J, Thompson J. Laryngopharyngeal sensory testing with modified barium swallow as predictors of aspiration pneumonia after stroke. *Laryngosc*. 1997;107:1254–1260.

Aviv JE, Sacco RL, Thomson J, et al. Silent laryngopharyngeal sensory deficits after stroke. *Ann Otol Rhinol Laryngol*. 1997;106:87–93.

Barohn, R. The therapeutic dilemma of inclusion body myositis. *Neurol*. 1997;48;567–568.

Baron BC, Dedo HH. Separation of the larynx and trachea for intractable aspiration. *Laryngosc*. 1980;90:1927–1932.

Barthelen W, Feussner H, Hanning CH, et al. Surgical therapy of Zenker's diverticulum: low risk and high efficiency. *Dysphagia*. 1990;5:13–19.

Bastian RW. Videoendoscopic evaluation of patients with dysphagia: an adjunct to the modified barrow swallow. *Otolaryngol Head Neck Surg*. 1991;104:339–350.

Bax, M. Terminology and classification of cerebral palsy. *Dev Med Child Neurol.* 1964;6:295–307.

Bielamowicz S, Berke GS, Gerratt BR. A comparison of Type I thyroplasty and arytenoid adduction. *J Voice.* 1995;9:466–472.

Blitzer A, Jahn AF, Deidar A. Semon's Law revisited: an electromyographic analysis of laryngeal synkinesis. *Ann Otol Rhinol Laryngol.* 1996;105:764–769.

Blonsky E, Logemann J, Boshes B. Comparison of speech and swallowing function in patients with tremor disorders and in normal geriatric patients: a cine fluorographic study. *J Gerontol.* 1975;30:299–305.

Brandenberg JH, Unger JM, Koschkee D. Vocal cord injection with autogenous fat: a long-term magnetic resonance imaging evaluation. *Laryngosc.* 1996;106:174–180.

Brasseur JG, Dodds WJ. Interpretation of intraluminal manometric measurements in terms of swallowing mechanics. *Dysphagia.* 1991;6:100–119.

Broniatowski M, Sonies BC, Rubin JS, Bradshaw CP, Spiegel JR, Bastian RW. *Otolaryngol Head Neck Surg.* 1999;120:464–473.

Brown KE. Peripheral consideration in improving obturator retention. *J Prosthet Dent.* 1968;20:176–181.

Bu'Lock F, Woolridge MW, Baum J D. Development of coordination of sucking, swallowing, and breathing: ultrasound study of term and preterm infants. *Dev Med Child Neurol.* 1990;32:669–678.

Capra NF. Mechanisms of oral sensation. *Dysphagia.* 1995;10:235–247.

Casas MJ, Kenny DJ, McPherson KA. Swallowing/ventilation interactions during oral swallow in normal children and children with cerebral palsy. *Dysphagia.* 1994;9:40–46.

Cichero JA, Hay G, Murdoch BE, Halley M. Videofluoroscopic fluids versus mealtime fluids: differences in viscosity and density made clear. *J Med Speech Lang Path.* 1997;5:203–215.

Condemi JJ. The autoimmune diseases. *JAMA.* 1992;268:2882–2892.

Cooper JS, Fu K, Marks J, Silverman S. Late effects of radiation therapy in the head and neck region. *Int J Radiat Oncol Biol Phys.* 1995;31:1141–1164.

Costantini M, Zaninotto G, Anselmino M, Marcon M, Iurilli V, Boccù C, Feltrin GP, Angelini C, Ancona E. Esophageal motor function in patients with myotonic dystrophy. *Dig Dis Sci.* 1996;41:2032–2038.

Crary MA. A direct intervention program for chronic neurogenic dysphagia secondary to brainstem stroke. *Dysphagia.* 1995;10:6–18.

Crary MA, Glowasky AL. Using botulinum toxin A to improve speech and swallowing function following total laryngectomy. *Arch Otolaryngol Head Neck Surg.* 1996;122:760–763.

Curran J, Groher ME. Development and dissemination of an aspiration risk reduction diet. *Dysphagia*. 1990;5:6–12.

Dahl M, Thommessen M, Rasmussen M, Selberg T. Feeding and nutritional characteristics in children with moderate to severe cerebral plasy. *Acta Paediatr*. 1996;85:697–701.

Dalakas, M. Immunopathogenesis of inflammatory myopathies. *Ann Neurol*. 1995;37:74–86.

Dantas RO, Kern MK, Massey BT, Dodds WJ, Kahrilas PJ, Brasseur JG, Cook IJ, Lang IM. Effect of swallowed bolus variables on the oral and pharyngeal phases of swallowing. *Am J Physiol*. 1990;258: G675–G681.

Dello Strologo L, Principato F, Sinibaldi D, Appiani AC, Terzi F, Dartois AM, Rizzoni G. Feeding dysfunction in infants with severe chronic renal failure after long-term nasogastric tube feeding. *Pediatr Nephrol*. 1997;11:84–86.

DePas WJ. Aspiration pneumonia. *Clin Chest Med*. 1991;12:269–284.

DePippo KL, Holas MA, Reding MJ. The Burke Dysphagia Screening Test: validation of its use in patients with stroke. *Arch Phys Med Rehabil*. 1994;75:1284–1286.

Dettelbach MA, Gross RD, Mahlmann J, Eibling DE. The effect of the Passy-Muir Valve on aspiration in patients with tracheostomy. *Head Neck*. 1995;17:297–302.

Dodds WJ, Logemann JA, Stewart ET. Radiologic assessment of abnormal oral and pharyngeal phases of swallowing. *Am J Roentgenol*. 1990;154:965–974.

Dulguerov P, Schweizer V, Caumel I, Esteve F. Medialization laryngoplasty. *Oto Head Neck Surg*. 1999;120:275–278.

Eibling DE, Snyderman CH, Eibling C. Laryngotracheal separation for intractable aspiration: a retrospective review of 34 patients. *Laryngosc*. 1995;105:83–85.

Feinberg MJ, Knebl J, Tully J. Prandial aspiration and pneumonia in an elderly population followed over 3 years. *Dysphagia*. 1996;11:104–109.

Field LH, Weiss CJ. Dysphagia with head injury. *Brain Inj*. 1989;3:19–26.

Fuh J-L, Lee R-C, Wang S-J, Lin C-H, Wang P-N, Chiang J-H, Liu H-C. Swallowing difficulty in Parkinson's disease. *Clin Neurol Neurosurg*. 1997;99:106–112.

Geterud A, Bake B, Bjelle A, Jonsson R, Sandberg N, Ejnell H. Swallowing problems in rheumatoid arthritis. *Acta Oto-Laryngologica*. 1991;111:1153–1161.

Hirano M, Kuroiwa Y, Tanaka S, Matsuoka H, Sato K. Dysphagia following various degrees of surgical resection for oral cancer. *Ann Otol Rhinol Laryngol*. 1992;101:138–141.

Horner J, Massey EW, Brazer SR. Aspiration in bilateral stroke patients. *Neurol.* 1990;40:1686–1688.

Hull MA, Rawlings J, Murray FE, et al. Audit of outcome of long-term enteral nutrition by percutaneous endoscopic gastrostomy. *Lancet.* 1993;341:869–872.

Huxley EJ, Viroslav J, Gray WR, et al. Pharyngeal aspiration in normal adults and patients with depressed consciousness. *Am J Med.* 1978;64:564–568.

Jaffe KM, McDonald CM, Ingman E, Haas J. Symptoms of upper gastrointestinal dysfunction in Duchenne muscular dystrophy: case-control study. *Arch Phys Med Rehabil.* 1990;71:742–744.

Jean A. Brainstem organization of the swallowing network. *Brain Behav Evolut.* 1984;25:109–116.

Johnson JT, Ferretti GA, Nethery WJ, Valdez IH, Fox PC, Ng D, Muscoplat CC, Gallagher SC. Oral pilocarpine for post-irradiation xerostomia in patients with head and neck cancer. *N Engl J Med.* 1993;329:390–395.

Kaplan S. Paralysis of deglutition, a post-poliomyelitis complication treated by section of the cricopharyngeus muscle. *Ann Surg.* 1951;133:572–573.

Kasarskis EJ, Berryman S, Vanderleest JG, Schneider AR, McClain CJ. Nutritional status of patients with amyotrophic lateral sclerosis: relation to the proximity of death. *Am J Clin Nutr.* 1996;63:130–137.

Kaye SA, Siraj QH, Agnew J, Hilson A, Black CM. Detection of early asymptomatic esophageal dysfunction in systemic sclerosis using a new scintigraphic grading method. *J Rheumatol.* 1996;23:297–301.

Kent RD, Kent JF, Weismer G, Sufit RL, Rosenbeck JC. Impairment of speech intelligibility in men with amyotrophic lateral sclerosis. *J Speech Hear Dis.* 1990;55:721–728.

Kirchner, JA. The motor activity of the cricopharyngeus muscle. *Laryngosc.* 1958;68:1119.

Koufman JA. The otolaryngologic manifestations of gastroesophageal reflux disease (GERD): a clinical investigation of 225 patients using ambulatory pH monitoring and an experimental investigation of the role of acid and pepsin in the development of laryngeal injury. *Laryngosc.* 1991;101:1–78.

Lang IM, Shaker R. Anatomy and physiology of the upper esophageal sphincter. *Am J Med.* 1997;103:50S–55S.

Langmore SE, Schatz K, Olsen N. Fibro-optic endoscopic examination of swallowing safety: a new procedure. *Dysphagia.* 1988;2:216–219.

Lazarus BA, Murphy JB, Culpepper L. Aspiration associated with long-term gastric versus jejunal feeding: a critical analysis of the literature. *Arch Phys Med Rehabil.* 1990;71:46–53.

Lazarus C, Logemann JA, Rademaker AW. Effects of bolus volume, viscosity, and repeated swallows in nonstroke subjects and stroke patients. *Arch Phys Med Rehabil.* 1993;74:1066–1070.

Leder SB. Effect of a one-way tracheostomy speaking valve on the incidence of aspiration in previously aspirating patients with tracheostomy. *Dysphagia.* 1999;14:73–77.

Leder SB, Tarro JM, Burrell MI. Effect of occlusion of a tracheostomy tube on aspiration. *Dysphagia.* 1996;11:254–258.

Leonard R, Gillis R. Effects of a prosthetic tongue on vowel intelligibility and food management in a patient with total glossectomy. *J Speech Hear Disord.* 1982;47:25–29.

Leopold NA, Kagel MC. Pharyngo-esophageal dysphagia in Parkinson's disease. *Dysphagia.* 1997;12:11–18.

Logemann J, Kahrilas PJ, Kobara M, Vakil N. The benefit of head rotation on pharyngoesophageal dysphagia. *Arch Phys Med Rehabil.* 1989;70:767–771.

Logemann J, Paulowski BR, Colagnelo L, Lazarus C, Fujiu M, Kahrilas PJ. Effects of a sour bolus on oropharyngeal swallowing measures in patients with neurogenic dysphagia. *J Speech Hear Res.* 1995;38:556–563.

Logemann JA, Rademaker AW, Paulowski BR, Kahrilas P. Effects of postural change on aspiration in head and neck surgical patients. *Otolaryngol Head Neck Surg.* 1994;110:222–227.

McConnel FMS, Hood D, Jackson K, O'Connor A. Analysis of intrabolus forces in patients with Zenker's diverticulum. *Laryngosc.* 1994;104:571–581.

Mehta PJ, Kosinski TF. Increased retention of a maxillary obturator prosthesis using osseointegrated intramobile cylinder dental implants: a clinical report. *J Prosthet Dent.* 1988;60:411.

Miller FR, Eliachar I. Managing the aspirating patient. *Am J Otolaryngol.* 1994;15:1–17.

Miller JL, Watkin KL. Lateral pharyngeal wall motion during swallowing using real time ultrasound. *Dysphagia.* 1997;12:125–132.

Mu L, Sanders I. The innervation of the human upper esophageal sphincter. *Dysphagia.* 1996;11:234–238.

Netterville JL, Jackson CG, Civantos FJ. Thyroplasty in the functional rehabilitation of neurotologic skull base surgery patients. *Am J Otolaryngol.* 1993;14:460–464.

Netterville JL, Korichak MJ, Winkle M, Courey MS, Ossoff RH. Vocal fold paralysis following the anterior approach to the cervical spine. *Ann Otol Rhinol Laryngol.* 1996;105:85–91.

Newall AR, Orser R, Hunt M. The control of oral secretions in bulbar ALS/MND. *J Neurol Sci.* 1996;139:43–44.

Newman LA, Cleveland RH, Blickman JG, Hillman RE, Jaramillo D. Videofluoroscopic analysis of the infant swallow. *Invest Radiol.* 1991;26:870–873.

Norton B, Homer W, Donnelley MT, et al. A randomized prospective comparison of percutaneous endoscopic gastrostomy and naso-gastric tube feeding after acute dysphagic stroke. *Lancet.* 1996;312:313–316.

Odderson IR, Keaton JC, McKenna BS. Swallow management in patients on an acute stroke pathway: quality is cost effective. *Arch Phys Med Rehabil.* 1995;76:1130–1133.

Oestreich AE, Dunbar JS. Pharyngonasal reflux; spectrum and signifi-cance in early childhood. *AJR.* 1984;141:924–925.

Olsson R, Nilsson H, Ekberg O. Simultaneous videoradiography and pharyngeal solid state manometry (videomanometry) in 25 nondys-phagic volunteers. *Dysphagia.* 1995;10:36–41.

Ott DJ, Chen YM, Hewson EG, et al. Esophageal motility: assessment with synchronous videofluoroscopy and manometry. *Radiol.* 1989; 173:419–422.

Palmer J, Rudin N, Lara G, Crompton A. Coordination of mastication and swallowing. *Dysphagia.* 1992;7:187–200.

Pardoe EM. Development of a multistage diet for dysphagia. *J Am Diet Assn.* 1993;93:568–571.

Périé S, Eymard B, Laccourreye L, Chaussade S, Fardeau M, Lacau St Guily J. Dysphagia in oculopharyngeal muscular dystrophy: a series of 22 French cases. *Neuromuscul Disord.* 1997;7:S96–S99.

Plaxico DT, Loughlin GM. Nasopharyngeal reflux and neonatal apnea, their relationship. *Am J Dis Child.* 1981;135:793–794.

Pou AM, Carrau RL, Eibling DE, Murry T. Laryngeal framework sur-gery for the management of aspiration in high vagal lesions. *Am Otolaryngol.* 1998;19:1–7.

Rasley A, Logemann JA, Kahrilas P, Rademaker AW, Pauloski B, Dodds WJ. Prevention of barium aspiration during videofluoroscopic swallowing studies: value of postural change. *Am J Roentgenol.* 1993;160:1005–1009.

Ren J, Shaker R, Lang I, Sui Z. Effect of volume, temperature and anes-thesia on the pharyngo-UES contractile reflex in humans. *Gastroen-terol.* 1995;108:A677.

Robbins J. Normal swallowing and aging. *Sem Neuro.* 1996;16:309–317.

Robbins J, Levine RL, Maser A, Rosenbek JC, Kempster GB. Swallow-ing after unilateral stroke of the cerebral cortex. *Arch Phys Med Reha-bil.* 1993;74:1295–1300.

Rogers BR, Arvedson J, Buck G, Smart P, Sall M. Characteristics of dys-phagia in children with cerebral palsy. *Dysphagia.* 1994;9:69–73.

Sasaki CT, Isaacson G. Functional anatomy of the larynx. *Clin N Amer.* 1988;21:595–612.

Sasaki CT, Suzuki M. Laryngeal reflexes in cat, dog, and man. *Arch Otolaryngol.* 1976;102:400.

Sasaki CT, Suzuki M, Horiuchi M, Kirchner JA. The effect of tracheostomy on the laryngeal closure reflex. *Laryngosc.* 1977;87:1428–1433.

Schatzki R, Gary JE. Dysphagia due to a diaphram-like localized narrowing in the lower esophagus. *Am J Roentgenol.* 1953;70:911–922.

Shaker R, Dodds WJ, Ren J, Hogan WJ, Arndorfer RC. Esophagoglottal closure reflex: a mechanism of airway protection. *Gastroenterol.* 1992;102:857–861.

Shaker R, Ren J, Hogan WJ, Liu J, Podvrsan B, Sui Z. Glottal function during postprandial gastroesophageal reflux. *Gastroenterol.* 1993;104:A581.

Shanahan TK, Logemann JA, Rademaker AW, Pauloski B, Kahrilas P. Chin down posture effects on aspiration in dysphagic patients. *Arch Phys Med Rehabil.* 1993;74:736–739.

Shapiro J, DeGirolami U, Martin S, Goyal R. Inflammatory myopathy causing pharyngeal dysphagia: a new entity. *Ann Otol Rhinol Laryngol.* 1996;105:331–335.

Shaw GY, Szewczyk MA, Searle J, Woodroof J. Autologous fat injection into the vocal folds: technical considerations and long-term follow-up. *Laryngosc.* 1997;107:100–186.

Slavitt H, Maragos NE. Physiologic assessment of arytenoid adduction. *Ann Otol Rhinol Laryngol.* 1992;101:312–317.

Sonies BC, Parent LJ, Morrish K, Baum BJ. Durational aspects of the oral-pharyngeal phase of swallow in normal adults. *Dysphagia.* 1988;3:1–10.

Stackler RJ, Hamlet SL, Choi J, Fleming S. Scintigraphic quantification of aspiration reduction with the Passy-Muir Valve. *Laryngosc.* 1996;106:231–234.

Strand EA, Miller RM, Yorkson KM, Hillel AD. Management of oral-pharyngeal dysphagia symptoms in amyotrophic lateral sclerosis. *Dysphagia.* 1996;11:129–139.

Stübgen JP. Limb girdle muscular dystrophy: a radiologic and manometric study of the pharynx and esophagus. *Dysphagia.* 1996;11:25–29.

Valles J, Artiguis A, Rello J, et al. Continuous aspiration of subglottic secretions in reventing ventilator-associated pneumonia. *Ann Int Med.* 1995;122:179–186.

van Overbeek JJM. Meditation on the pathogenesis of hypopharyngeal (Zenker's) diverticulum and a report of endoscopic treatment in 545 patients. *Ann Otol Rhinol Laryngol.* 1994;103:178–185.

Waterman ET, Koltai PJ, Downey JC, Cacace AT. Swallowing disorders in a population of children with cerebral palsy. *Int J Pediatr Otorhinolaryngol.* 1992;24:63–71.

Weber F, Woolridge M, Baum J. An ultrasonographic study of the organization of sucking and swallowing by newborn infants. *Dev Med Child Neurol.* 1996;28:19–24.

Weissman JL. Corkscrew esophagus. *Am J Otolaryngol.* 1993;14:53–54.

Willig TN, Paulus J, Saint Guly JL, Beon C, Navarro J. *Arch Phys Med Rehabil.* 1994;75:1175–1181.

Wilson S, Thach BB, Brouilette R, Abu-Osba Y. Coordination of breathing and swallowing in human infants. *J Appl Physiol.* 1981;50:851–858.

Woodson GE. Configuration of the glottis in laryngeal paralysis I: clinical study. *laryngosc.* 1993;103:1227–1234.

Woodson GE: Cricopharyngeal myotomy and arytenoid adduction in the management of combined laryngeal and pharyngeal paralysis. *Otolaryngol HNS.* 1997;116:339–343.

Yin S, Qui W, Strucker F. Major patterns of laryngeal electromyography and their clinical applications. *Laryngosc.* 1997;107:126–136.

References-Book Chapters

Alberts MJ, Roses AD. Myotonic muscular dystrophy. *Neurol Clin.* 1989;7:1–8.

Buckwalter JA, Sasaki CT. Effect of tracheotomy on laryngeal function. *Otolaryngol Clin North Am.* 1984;17:41–48.

Fox RI. Sjögren's syndrome. In: Kelley WN, Harris ED, Ruddy S, Sledge CB, eds. *Textbook of Rheumatology.* Philadelphia, Pa: W.B. Saunders Company; 1997:955–968.

Gesell A, Amatruda CS. *Developmental Diagnosis: Normal and Abnormal Child Development.* 2nd ed. New York: Paul H. Hoeber Inc.; 1956.

Logemann JA. Therapy for oropharyngeal swallowing disorders. In: Perlman AL, Schulze-Delrieu K, eds. *Deglutition and Its Disorders.* San Diego, Calif: Singular Publishing Group; 1997:449–462.

Logemann J. Speech and swallowing rehabilitation for head and neck tumor patients. In: Myers EN, Suen J, eds. *Cancer of the Head and Neck.* 2nd ed. New York: Churchill Livingston; 1997:1021–1043.

Niederman MS, Fein AM. Pneumonia in the elderly. *Geriatr Clin North Am.* 1986;2:241–268.

Reynolds JC, Parkman HP. Achalasia *Gastroenterol Clin N Am.* 1989;18:223–255.

Seibold JR. Scleroderma. In: Kelley WN, Harris ED, Ruddy S, Sledge CB, eds. *Textbook of Rheumatology.* 5th ed. Philadelphia Pa: W.B. Saunders Company; 1997:1133–1162.

Sekul E, Dalakas M. Inclusion body myositis: new concepts. *Semin Neurol.* 1993;13:256–263.

References—Books

Carrau RL, Murry T, eds. *Comprehensive Management of Swallowing Disorders.* San Diego, Calif: Singular Publishing Group; 1999.

Groher ME. *Dysphagia: Diagnosis and Management.* Stoneham, Mass: Butterworth, 1984.

Hockabee ML, Pelletier CA. *Management of Adult Neurogenic Dysphagia.* San Diego, Calif: Singular Publishing Group; 1998.

Leonard R, Kendall K. *Dysphagia Assessment and Treatment Planning: A Team Approach.* San Diego, Calif: Singular Publishing Group; 1998.

Logemann J. *Evaluation and Treatment of Swallowing Disorders.* San Antonio, Tex: Pro Ed; 1993.

Martin JH. The somatic sensory system. In: Martin JH, ed. *Neuroanatomy; Text and Atlas.* New York: Elsevier; 1989: 122–123.

Miller AJ. The Neuroscientific Principles of Swallowing and Dysphagia. San Diego, Calif: Singular Publishing Group; 1998.

Perlman AL, Rosenthal JJ, Sheppard M, Lotze W, eds. *Dysphagia and the Child With Developmental Disabilities: Medical, Clinical, and Family Interventions.* San Diego, Calif: Singular Publishing Group; 1997:1–4.

Perlman AL, Schulze-Delrieu K, eds. *Deglutition and Its Disorders.* San Diego, Calif: Singular Publishing Group; 1997:449–462.

Sullivan PA, Guilford AM. *Swallowing Intervention in Oncology.* San Diego, Calif: Singular Publishing Group; 1998.

Index

Squamous cell carcinoma, 8
Sticky property, 154
Stomatitis, 46
Strain, 152
Strokes, 5–7, 30, 86, 166
Structural anatomy, 83
Super-supraglottic swallow, 127
Supraglottic swallow, 127
Surgical treatment of swallowing
   disorders. *See* Treatment of
   swallowing disorders, surgical
Swallow maneuvers, 126–129
Swallow postures, 129–131
Swallowing center, 21–22
Swallowing disorders, 25–63
   aspiration pneumonia, 27–30
   autoimmune diseases, 30–34
   conditions that lead to, 10
   critical care patients, 35–36
   esophageal, 36–44
   infectious diseases, 44–45
   medications that cause, 46–49
   neoplasms, 49–50
   neurologic/neuromuscular, 50–61
   and radiation therapy, 61–62
   see also Treatment of swallowing
      disorders
Swallowing function, 13–23
   central neural control, 21–23
   components of, 14
   diagnosis of dysphagia according
      to phases of, 18–19
   esophageal phase, 18–19
   oral phase, 16–17
   oral preparatory phase, 15–16
   pharyngeal phase, 17
   sphincters/valves, 19–21
Swallowing severity scale, 53
Systemic lupus erythematosus
   (SLE), 34

T cells, 30
Teflon® injection, 136–137
Tegretol®, 49
Temporal arteritis, 31

Temporo-mandibular joint (TMJ)
   syndrome, 32–33
Texture, 154–159
Therabite®, 119
Thermal stimulation, 122
Thickeners, 151, 154, 160
Thinning agents, 154
Thioridazine, 49
Thorazine®, 49
TMJ syndrome. *See* Temporo-
   mandibular joint
Tongue, 15–17
Tongue base, 69
Tongue and mandible exercises,
   119, 121
Tonsils, 69
Tracheal aspiration, 92
Tracheostomy, 72–75, 145–147
   airway pressure changes, 73
   cricothyrotomy, 147
   decannulation, 147
   expiratory speaking valves, 73–74
   expiratory valves, 146–147
   fenestrated tracheostomy tube,
      146–147
   glottic closure, 74–75
   laryngeal elevation, 74
   pharyngeal transit, 75
   physiological changes
      following, 73
   recommendations for, 145–146
Transducer, 98
Transfer phase, 15
Transverse tongue response, 83
Traumatic brain injury, 61
Treatment of swallowing disorders
   nonsurgical
      approaches to, 113
      dentition and mastication, 114
      head-raising exercise, 122–123
      lingual prostheses, 116, 118
      methods summary, 131
      oral motor exercises, 119–125
      palatal lowering prostheses,
         114–116
      soft palate prostheses, 116–117
      studies of, 126–127